Quick and Delicious

Weeknight 10-Minute Dinners Cookbook: 250 Quick & Tasty Meals for Busy People with Just 3 Ingredients

Evelyn Anderson

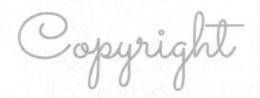

Table of Contents

Chapter 2

15-MINUTE Recipes 43

Chapter 3
20-MINUTE Recipes 79

Chapter 4

30-MINUTE Recipes 115

Quick and Delicious

Bonus Section

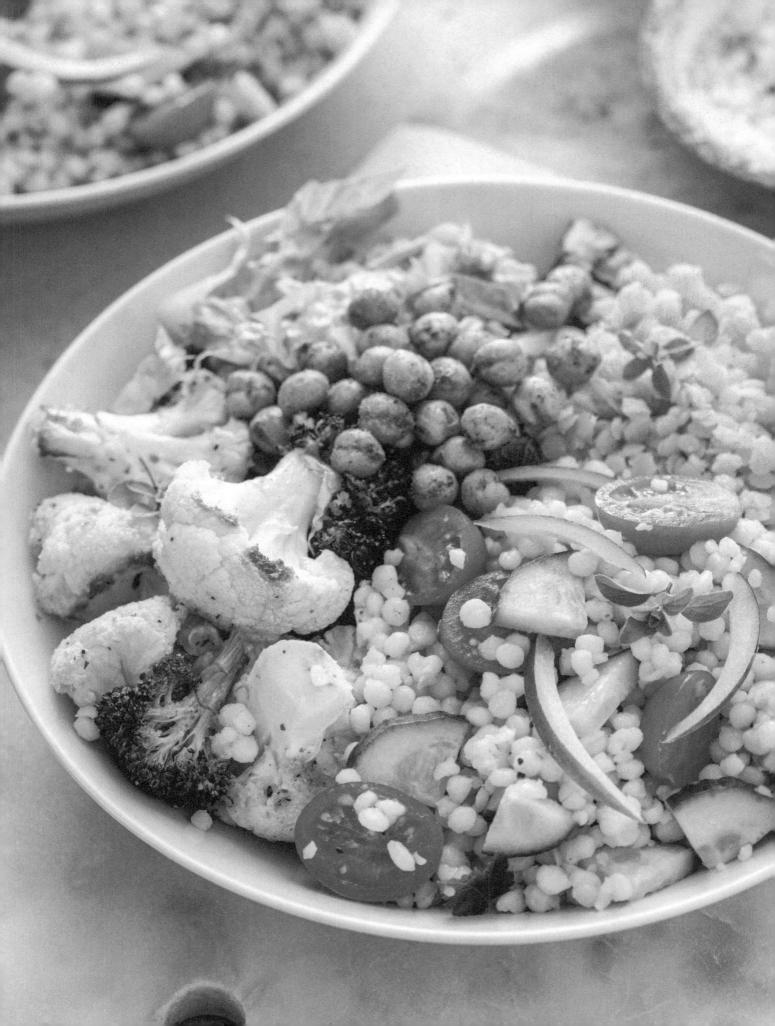

Introduction

Welcome to Quick and Delicious Weeknight Dinners

Welcome to Quick and Delicious Weeknight Dinners, a cookbook designed to make meal preparation fast, simple, and satisfying for everyone, even on the busiest nights. In this book, you'll discover 250 recipes tailored for people with packed schedules who still want to enjoy healthy and delicious meals at home. Every recipe here is crafted with just three key ingredients—no lengthy shopping lists or elaborate steps. With simplicity at its core, this book helps you transform a handful of everyday ingredients into nourishing meals. You won't need to hunt down specialty items; everything you'll need is likely already in your pantry or fridge, ready to be turned into something delightful.

This book is organized by preparation time, giving you control over your time in the kitchen. For days when you're rushed and need to keep things extra short, explore the "Truly 10-Minute Recipes" section. Here, you'll find recipes that deliver flavor and satisfaction without taking up more than ten minutes of your time, ideal for those hectic days. If you have a little more time, turn to the "15-Minute Recipes," where you'll find dishes that allow for a bit more creativity while still keeping your time commitment low. When you're in the mood for something more substantial but want to stay efficient, the "20-Minute Recipes" section will be your go-to, offering hearty and filling meals that come together quickly. Finally, the "30-Minute Recipes" round out the selection with options that may require a few extra minutes but are still swift enough to fit into any weeknight and are perfect for a cozy, satisfying dinner.

Each recipe is designed for convenience and versatility, making it easy to adapt based on what's on hand. With these simple, three-ingredient combinations, you'll quickly see how easy it is to make mealtime stress-free and enjoyable. To get started, here's what you'll need: just a few essential kitchen tools—typically, a pan, a pot, and a handful of utensils like a knife and a spatula. These tools will take you from breakfast to dinner, allowing you to create all 250 recipes with minimal cleanup. Each recipe has clear, step-by-step instructions, so you'll feel confident creating each dish even if you're not an experienced cook.

There are also extra goods in this book to make your cooking even more accessible and additional fun. Beginning with a custom-crafted, downloadable shopping list to streamline your grocery trips and reduce anxiety. The list is made up of the essential flavorings most used in it, so you can go buy them and have everything to cook at all times, such as a homemade fast dish. Also included is a chapter on how to stock your budget-friendly pantry. The ingredients are versatile for reuse across multiple recipes or non-perishable to decrease waste and budget. With this strategy, you can utilize as much of your grocery haul as possible without having many obscure things that are very expensive and you would only use for one or two dishes.

For an even better cooking experience, each recipe is accompanied by a video that demonstrates visually how it should be done, including videos of fast & loose demonstrations. Anyone can understand these quick, easy to follow demos, making the book for Any Skill level. These videos are designed to give you the extra confidence you need, whether you are a novice or an experienced home cook. A step-by-step along the way to make you feel, like me, that there is your own personal cooking teacher in my kitchen.

Perhaps most importantly, this book has been created with an eye to readers on the broader world, and so it features a helpful unit conversion chart. Each recipe in the book has a dedicated page that converts all American measurements to their metric counterparts so you can cook anywhere without unnecessary difficulty. Ounces to grams, cups, and milliliters — this guide provides the answer in one handy chart.

So now that you have an idea of what to expect from this book, let us jump into the recipes and find out how easy it is for everyone who reads my book. After a long day of work, you walk in the door and take one glance into your pantry before whipping something nourishing up without even batting an eyelid. Every recipe in this book equals a new way to make meal time easier and more teasing for you, your friends, and your family today. No more weeknight stress in the kitchen or days on end of takeout. Quick and Delicious Weeknight Dinners has what you need to make any night less of a hassle and more fun at the table, with dishes that are sure to please!

How to Use This Book

This is a book to slot into your life, choosing to depend on whichever moment you have (or don't) and whichever meal you want (or don't). Recipes are arranged by prep time, so you can find exactly what you're in the mood for in seconds, whether it be a snack, light meal, or full dinner. Keeping in mind the busy schedules, every recipe in this book uses a maximum of 3 main ingredients. With these everyday ingredients, which you probably already have in your pantry or fridge, meal prep can be simple, fast, and stress-free.

The first section, titled Truly 10-Minute Recipes, is designed for those moments when time is tight and you need a meal in under ten minutes. These recipes are perfect for when you're racing against the clock or just looking to get something on the table quickly. Even though the preparation is brief, these meals still provide all the flavor and satisfaction you'd expect from a home-cooked dish. From hearty breakfasts to energize your day to quick lunches and light dinners, the 10-minute recipes make use of simple techniques and minimal cooking time. Expect options like Avocado and Egg Toast, Grilled Cheese Sandwich, and Tuna Salad. These are ideal when you want something fresh and tasty without spending too much time in the kitchen.

The 15-Minute Recipes section is a bit of a step up, allowing a few more minutes but still providing for the busy schedule. Ideally, these meals work for days that are a touch less frenetic or maybe a Saturday afternoon when you need a bit more diversity. In fifteen minutes, you will be establishing meals that seem far more substantive, along with flavors and styles that go above the fundamentals. There are recipes such as Chicken Alfredo Pasta, Turkey Meatballs with Marinara, and Shrimp Fajitas being published here. Those extra five minutes are out of convenience, so even if you have a bit more time for creativity (and we mean this in the best possible way), these recipes can still be made simply.

Finally, A section of 20-Minute Recipes provides ideas for hearty main dishes with additional seasoning and unique ingredient combinations. This twenty-minute meal gives you a little more layering of flavors and a few more involved techniques, but the prep and cook time on this is still pretty quick. These meals are perfect for those evenings when you want something a little heartier or when you're cooking for the entire family. These include Chicken Parmesan, Spaghetti with Meat Sauce, and Shrimp Tacos with Avocado, all designed to deliver delectable meals without taking hours from your day. This part allows you to play around a little more and get a completely satisfying meal that does not feel rushed.

The last part with the recipes is called 30-Minute Recipes, which I save for when you have slightly more time and are craving a more substantial and indulgent recipe. Each dish provides variety in flavor and texture but still sits within the quick category as far as cooking goes —these recipes keep everyone happy. With thirty minutes to work with, we have some more options — more elaborate techniques, more complex flavors, and bigger servings. These recipes can be used for dinner as a family, entertaining guests, or treating yourself to a bit of a stop and smell the roses meal. Whether you're cooking Chicken Cacciatore or Thai Green Curry or Beef Stir-Fry with Veggies, these options will elevate any meal to exceptional occasion levels — even on a weeknight.

To make your cooking experience as effortless as pleasing, every section in this book has been arranged very systematically. From a speedy meal in the 10-minute section to giving yourself some time to prepare a 30-minute recipe, they strike the right balance between nutrition and flavor for you. Each recipe is written in an easy, non-jargon-filled way, so you won't waste time trying to decode the instructions. It's not a complicated cooking language, so even if you are not a talented chef, you will be quite at home with each step.

Every meal is structured to be adaptable as well. If you find yourself with an extra ingredient or two, feel free to enhance the recipes with your own touch. This book encourages a relaxed, creative approach to cooking, where you can modify and adjust the recipes to suit your preferences or dietary needs. The three-ingredient base is meant to simplify and speed up your time in the kitchen, but the recipes are also designed to be flexible so that you can personalize each dish however you like.

Perfect Meals for Busy People is the ideal cookbook for you whether you are a busy professional, a time-pressed parent, or just someone who appreciates a quick, delicious meal. It's about bringing ease, fun, and joy to your daily cooking rather than drudgery. Select recipes depending on how much time you have at your disposal, and you will find time to prepare home-cooked meals for your family, no matter how loaded your schedule is. This method takes away the burden of cooking, makes it a convenient and satisfying process, and gets you eating healthy food without breaking a sweat.

We always say that cooking for yourself — when you have the time — is an act of self-care, and with this book, you can weave it into your regular routine. Make each of these sections — from the shortest recipes to the heaviest — a place where you can find your love for cooking even when you may be working within a limited time frame. These recipes will let you sit down to Good Food every day — without putting stress on lengthy prep time or multistep, sophisticated processes, turning weeknight dinners from a task to a treat.

What You'll Need

In order to keep things as simple as possible, the recipes in this book use only basic kitchen tools. Forget pulling out your arsenal of gadgets: we designed these recipes so you can enjoy delicious, hearty meals using minimal tools. What this implies is that you will not require any complex apparatus; rather, you will only depend on a couple of key things that the majority of kitchens already possess. The idea is to make it really simple and fun to cook, reduce cooking time and clean up time so that when you want to treat yourself to a good meal, it's as easy as pie.

The must have equipment to have on hand would be a trustworthy pan, a multipurpose pot, and a handful of utensils. With these, you will be equipped to make every recipe in the book. A high-quality skillet can be used for a variety of tasks — if you need to whip a bunch of veggies for a quick sauté, sear some chicken, or make a stir-fry, this is the go-to tool. Choose one that is uniformly heated to retain consistency in terms of cooking and the taste delivered to your meals. In fact, for the easiest recipes, a non-stick pan is ideal as oil input is minimized and cleaning is faster.

Second, a good-sized pot is also important. You will use this pot a lot for tasks that will include boiling pasta, soups, stews, and even one-pot meals. Since a good portion of the recipes in this book ask for just three ingredients, a medium-sized pot is generally the right size. This should not be anything too big and cumbersome; you need something functional, something that will fit nicely on the stove and be easy enough to handle. Having a lid for your pot is a plus, as that will help reduce the cooking times and keep your foods warm if you are preparing more than one serving.

Only a few things are essential when it comes to utensils. A good chef's knife is needed for preparing and chopping most food, and a small paring knife may also be handy when slicing fruits or peeling vegetables. A sharp knife is a fast and safe knife, and every slice will be neat and quick, which is why you should always keep your knives sharpened. A durable yet easy-to-clean cutting board is necessary, too, in addition to a proper knife. Get a gigantic board to prepare or chop multiple ingredients at once without switching between the boards.

A spatula is also one of the best tools for flipping, stirring, and cooking ingredients evenly. For scrambled eggs, grilled sandwiches, or pan-seared meats, a flexible spatula is key for effective sliding on and off the heat without sticking or tearing. Silicone or rubber spatulas are soft on non-stick surfaces and can heat resist very high temperatures, so we can use them for multiple cooking tasks.

Also, measuring tools are handy, but tons of these recipes lend themselves well to making them not super precise. For a more accurate point of reference, a measuring cup and spoons come in handy when you need to use things like pasta, grains, or spices. That said, these are forgiving recipes, so feel free to eyeball measurements as needed or adjust amounts to your taste (always!), which is part of the fun of cooking and why this book is designed to give you that freedom.

A few other small items that help with cooking are also included. If you want to flip food or otherwise handle hot food safely, tongs are great, and a ladle is perfect for when spooning soup or stew. A cheese grater comes in handy for recipes that require grated cheese or zest, but it is not necessary. These extra tools are mostly optional, and you can easily swap them for utensils you already have in your kitchen. These recipes are perfect because you can make them fit what you have in your kitchen.

This will make cooking more enjoyable, as you will find it a more achievable activity as long as you focus on these simple yet versatile tools. You don't need an elaborate setup or fancy appliances; just a few essentials will help you prepare meals that are satisfying, nutritious, and full of fresh flavors. This method allows you to get cooking quickly and efficiently and allows for easy cleanup. Food prep is not an ordeal, and with a few implements close at hand, your circumstances need never resemble that.

This also implies that you can whip these up wherever you find yourself, whether in a fully equipped kitchen or a basic provision. Recipes that honor real-life — practical recipes, easy to prepare. Given a handful of tools and a little love, you'll find yourself customizing every recipe in the way that only a home cook discovering her rhythm can have during even the most hectic of days. The goal of this book is to make cooking feel easy and fun so that every time you enter the kitchen, you are ready to whip up something delicious without fuss.

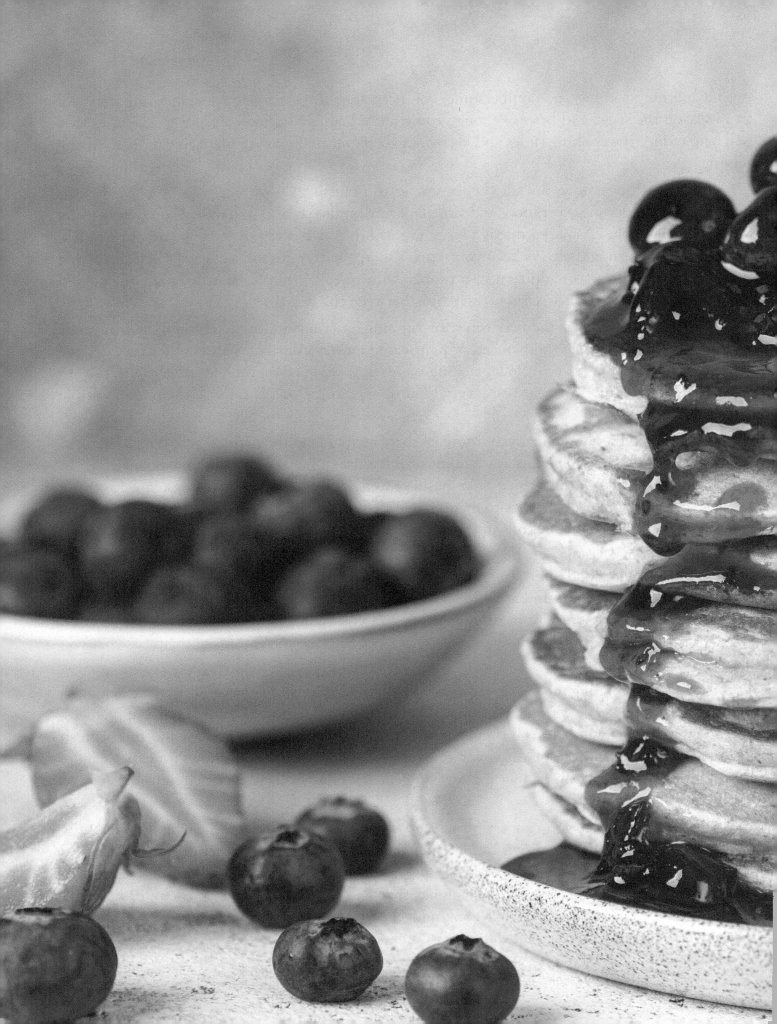

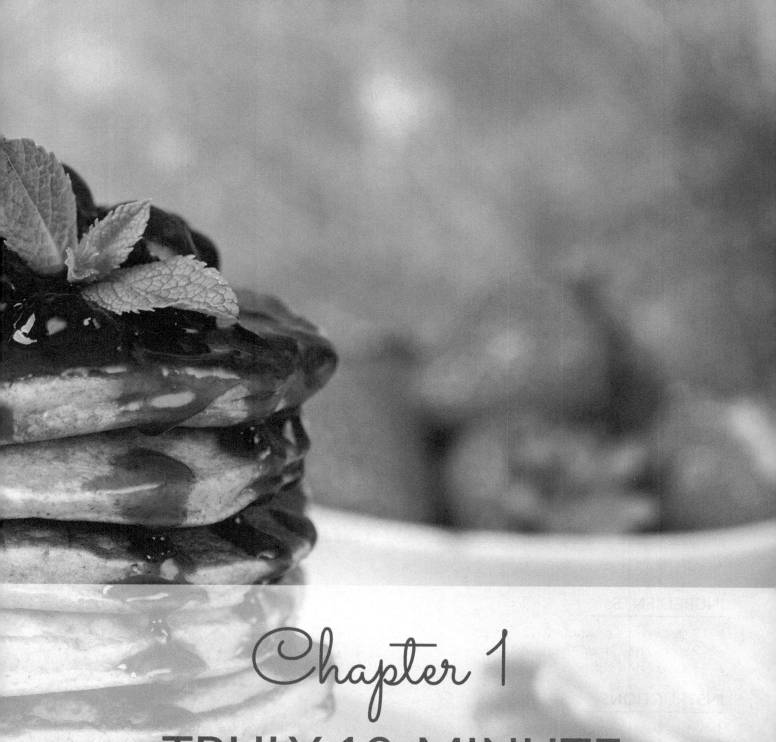

Chapter 1
TRULY 10-MINUTE
Recipes

These recipes are guaranteed to be ready in under 10 minutes.

Avocado and Egg Toast

 Under 10 minutes

INGREDIENTS:

- » 1 slice whole-grain bread, toasted
- » ½ ripe avocado, mashed
- » 1 large egg, cooked to preference (poached, fried, or scrambled)

INSTRUCTIONS:

1. Bake the bread until it is a golden brown coloration.
2. When the bread is toasting put the avocado in a little bowl and mash with a fork then sprinkle with the pinch of salt if you so desire.
3. Top the toast with the mashed avocado ensuring that it is spread to your desired thickness.
4. Cover with the cooked egg, and dust with a few of pepper or red pepper flakes to taste.

NUTRITIONAL VALUES (PER SERVING):

Calories: 220; Protein: 8g; Carbohydrates: 18g; Fiber: 6g; Total Fat: 14g

Grilled Cheese Sandwich

 Under 10 minutes

INGREDIENTS:

- » 2 slices white or whole-wheat bread
- » 2 slices cheddar or American cheese
- » 1 tablespoon butter

INSTRUCTIONS:

1. Make sure to spread the butter on one of the surfaces of each of those slices of breads.
2. Set a nonstick skillet on the 2nd ring of heat and put one slice of bread in the pan with the buttered side down.
3. Layer the cheese slices on top of the bread, then place the second bread slice on top, buttered side up.
4. Cook for 3-4 minutes on each side, pressing down slightly with a spatula, until the bread is golden brown and the cheese is fully melted.

NUTRITIONAL VALUES (PER SERVING):

Calories: 330; Protein: 10g; Carbohydrates: 28g; Fiber: 2g; Total Fat: 20g

Scrambled Eggs with Spinach

 Under 10 minutes

INGREDIENTS:

» 2 large eggs, beaten
» 1/2 cup fresh spinach, chopped
» 1 tablespoon butter or olive oil

INSTRUCTIONS:

1. In a nonstick skillet over medium heat, melt the butter or add olive oil.
2. Add the chopped spinach and sauté for about 1 minute until the leaves begin to soften.
3. Pour in the beaten eggs, gently stirring to combine with the spinach.
4. Stirring for further 2-3minutes so that the eggs chanced to your preferred preferability. It is best enjoyed warm and this recipe will serve you healthy breakfast that will kick start your day in the mornings.

NUTRITIONAL VALUES (PER SERVING):

Calories: 200; Protein: 12g; Carbohydrates: 2g; Fiber: 1g; Total Fat: 16g

Chicken Lettuce Wraps

 Under 10 minutes

INGREDIENTS:

» Chicken breast 58 g, cooked and shredded drained weight
» 4 large lettuce leaves preferably using romaine or butter lettuce.
» 2 tablespoons hoisin sauce

INSTRUCTIONS:

1. Spread the lettuce leaves and now portion the shredded chicken for the lettuce wrap.
2. This will remind you of the sauces used in Chinese cooking; pour about half a tablespoon of hoisin sauce on every portion of the chicken.
3. Make a hand held wrap by encasing the filling in each lettuce leaf through rolling or wrapping it gently.
4. Best eaten fresh as soon as assembled, this is a perfect light snack or meal.

NUTRITIONAL VALUES (PER SERVING):

Calories: 150; Protein: 14g; Carbohydrates: 4g; Fiber: 1g; Total Fat: 8g

Quick Tuna Salad

 Under 10 minutes

INGREDIENTS:

» 1 can tuna in water, drained (5 oz)
» 2 tablespoons mayonnaise
» 1 celery stalk, finely chopped

INSTRUCTIONS:

1. In a mixing bowl, combine the drained tuna, mayonnaise, and chopped celery.
2. Use a fork to mix the ingredients, breaking up any larger tuna chunks until the mixture is smooth and well combined.
3. Serve the tuna salad as a filling for sandwiches, over a bed of greens, or with crackers for a quick, protein-packed snack.

NUTRITIONAL VALUES (PER SERVING):

Calories: 220; Protein: 20g; Carbohydrates: 2g; Fiber: 0g; Total Fat: 14g

Veggie Stir-Fry

 Under 10 minutes

INGREDIENTS:

» 1 cup mixed bell peppers, sliced
» 1 small zucchini, sliced
» 1 tablespoon soy sauce

INSTRUCTIONS:

1. Turn burner to medium-high heat and place the skillet that is safe for a non-stick cookware. Put the sliced bell peppers and zucchini.
2. I also used the Wok for this reason because the vegetables should be stir frequently so that they will not stick on the bottom of the pan and at the same time be cooked evenly.
3. Lastly, pour the soy sauce over the veggies and allow the food sauté for another 3-5 minutes, until the vegetables are crisp tender.
4. It is best presented as a side dish and it can also be eaten over rice if you want a light meal.

NUTRITIONAL VALUES (PER SERVING):

Calories: 80; Protein: 2g; Carbohydrates: 12g; Fiber: 3g; Total Fat: 2g

Pasta with Garlic and Olive Oil

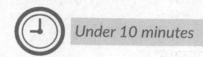 *Under 10 minutes*

INGREDIENTS:

» 1 cup cooked pasta (spaghetti or linguine)
» 2 tablespoons olive oil
» 2 garlic cloves, thinly sliced

INSTRUCTIONS:

1. Heat the olive oil in a skillet with medium flame. Put the garlic slices in and stir for 1-2 minutes until crispy and fragrant but can turn black easily.
2. Place the cooked pasta into the skillet and coat it with the garlic infused oil available.
3. Season it with salt and pepper which may suit your taste bud then transfer it another plate. Serve it straight away with a spoon, further garnish with more red pepper flakes or Para s with some grated parmesan cheese on top.

NUTRITIONAL VALUES (PER SERVING):

Calories: 300; Protein: 6g; Carbohydrates: 40g; Fiber: 2g; Total Fat: 12g

Tomato and Mozzarella Salad

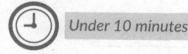 *Under 10 minutes*

INGREDIENTS:

» 1 cup cherry tomatoes, halved
» ½ cup fresh mozzarella, cubed
» 1 tablespoon balsamic vinegar

INSTRUCTIONS:

1. Take a medium bowl and add the cherries tomatoes which is halved and mozzarella which is cut into cubes. Turn from side to side to ensure that all the constituents are well combined.
2. It is then advisable to shower the apricot glaze very gently over the slices of tomato and mozzarella.
3. Then sprinkling a pinch of salt and pepper, before stirring gently. Pleasantly served immediately preferably complimented with basil leaves to boost the freshness of the dish. This salad is best eaten with grilled meats or can be used as an appetiser.

NUTRITIONAL VALUES (PER SERVING):

Calories: 150; Protein: 8g; Carbohydrates: 7g; Fiber: 1g; Total Fat: 10g

Spinach and Feta Omelette

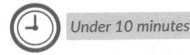 *Under 10 minutes*

INGREDIENTS:

» 2 large eggs, beaten
» ¼ cup fresh spinach, chopped
» 2 tablespoons feta cheese, crumbled

INSTRUCTIONS:

1. Heat a nonstick skillet over medium heat and pour in the beaten eggs, swirling to cover the pan's surface evenly.
2. Sprinkle the chopped spinach and crumbled feta cheese over one side of the omelette.
3. Cook for 2-3 minutes until the eggs are set, then carefully fold the omelette in half. Transfer to a plate and serve warm. This dish is great for a nutritious breakfast or a light lunch.

NUTRITIONAL VALUES (PER SERVING):

Calories: 200; Protein: 12g; Carbohydrates: 2g; Fiber: 1g; Total Fat: 16g

Chicken Breast with Lemon

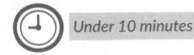 *Under 10 minutes*

INGREDIENTS:

» 1 boneless, skinless chicken breast
» 1 tablespoon olive oil
» Juice of ½ lemon

INSTRUCTIONS:

1. Season the chicken breast lightly with salt and pepper. In a skillet over medium heat, add the olive oil and heat until shimmering.
2. Place the chicken in the skillet and cook for 3-4 minutes on each side until golden and cooked through.
3. Squeeze the lemon juice over the chicken, allowing it to absorb the citrus flavor. Serve immediately, garnished with lemon zest or fresh herbs if desired. This simple, flavorful dish is perfect for a quick dinner.

NUTRITIONAL VALUES (PER SERVING):

Calories: 250; Protein: 26g; Carbohydrates: 1g; Fiber: 0g; Total Fat: 15g

Instant Tomato Soup

 Under 10 minutes

INGREDIENTS:

» 1 cup tomato juice
» ¼ cup heavy cream
» Salt and pepper to taste

INSTRUCTIONS:

1. In a saucepan over medium heat, pour in the tomato juice and stir in the heavy cream. Stir continuously to combine the ingredients smoothly.
2. Heat the mixture for 5-7 minutes, stirring occasionally until it's warmed through and slightly thickened.
3. Season with salt and pepper to taste, adjusting as desired. Serve immediately in a bowl, optionally garnished with fresh basil or a sprinkle of grated Parmesan for extra flavor. This quick, creamy soup is perfect as a cozy meal starter.

NUTRITIONAL VALUES (PER SERVING):

Calories: 150; Protein: 2g; Carbohydrates: 6g; Fiber: 1g; Total Fat: 12g

Pancakes with Berries

 Under 10 minutes

INGREDIENTS:

» 1 cup pancake mix
» ¾ cup water
» ½ cup mixed berries (blueberries, strawberries, raspberries)

INSTRUCTIONS:

1. In a mixing bowl, combine the pancake mix and water, stirring until the batter is smooth and free of lumps.
2. Heat a nonstick skillet over medium heat, and pour batter to create small pancakes.
3. Cook each side for 2-3 minutes or until bubbles appear and the edges are golden. Serve topped with fresh mixed berries for a burst of natural sweetness and a touch of color.

NUTRITIONAL VALUES (PER SERVING):

Calories: 200; Protein: 5g; Carbohydrates: 32g; Fiber: 3g; Total Fat: 5g

Shrimp and Avocado Salad

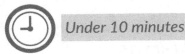 *Under 10 minutes*

INGREDIENTS:

» ½ cup cooked shrimp, peeled and chopped
» ½ avocado, diced
» 1 tablespoon lime juice

INSTRUCTIONS:

1. In a medium bowl, combine the cooked shrimp and diced avocado.
2. Drizzle the lime juice over the shrimp and avocado, and gently toss to coat.
3. Season with a little salt and beaten black pepper then, serve immediately. This salad can easily be enjoyed on the side or consumed as a light, simple lunch. It goes well with a piece of whole grain bread, lettuce or other greens.

NUTRITIONAL VALUES (PER SERVING):

Calories: 180; Protein: 12g; Carbohydrates: 8g; Fiber: 4g; Total Fat: 12g

Veggie Wrap with Hummus

 Under 10 minutes

INGREDIENTS:

» 1 whole wheat tortilla
» 2 tablespoons hummus
» ½ cup mixed veggies (carrot sticks, bell pepper strips, cucumber slices)

INSTRUCTIONS:

1. Spread the hummus evenly across the tortilla, ensuring even coverage for flavor in every bite.
2. Layer the mixed vegetables on top of the hummus, distributing them evenly.
3. Roll up the tortilla tightly, slice in half, and serve immediately. This quick veggie wrap makes a nutritious snack or light meal. For added flavor, you can sprinkle in some herbs or a dash of hot sauce.

NUTRITIONAL VALUES (PER SERVING):

Calories: 190; Protein: 6g; Carbohydrates: 30g; Fiber: 5g; Total Fat: 7g

Egg Fried Rice

 Under 10 minutes

INGREDIENTS:

- » 1 cup cooked rice
- » 1 large egg, beaten
- » 1 tablespoon soy sauce

INSTRUCTIONS:

1. In a skillet over medium heat, add the cooked rice, stirring occasionally to prevent sticking.
2. Push the rice to one side of the skillet and pour in the beaten egg, scrambling it until fully cooked.
3. Mix the scrambled egg with the rice, then add the soy sauce and stir well to combine. Serve warm, garnished with green onions if desired. This dish is perfect as a light meal or side dish.

NUTRITIONAL VALUES (PER SERVING):

Calories: 210; Protein: 7g; Carbohydrates: 34g; Fiber: 1g; Total Fat: 5g

Sautéed Zucchini with Parmesan

 Under 10 minutes

INGREDIENTS:

- » 1 small zucchini, thinly sliced
- » 1 tablespoon olive oil
- » 1 tablespoon grated Parmesan cheese

INSTRUCTIONS:

1. In a skillet, heat the olive oil over medium heat, then add the zucchini slices in an even layer.
2. Sauté the zucchini for 3-4 minutes until they're tender and slightly golden.
3. Sprinkle with Parmesan cheese, season with salt and pepper, and serve warm. This quick and savory dish is perfect as a side or light snack, offering both flavor and nutrition.

NUTRITIONAL VALUES (PER SERVING):

Calories: 110; Protein: 2g; Carbohydrates: 5g; Fiber: 1g; Total Fat: 9g

Grilled Salmon with Asparagus

 Under 10 minutes

INGREDIENTS:

» 4 oz salmon fillet
» 1 cup asparagus spears, trimmed
» 1 tablespoon olive oil

INSTRUCTIONS:

1. Brush the salmon fillet and asparagus with olive oil, and season with salt and pepper.
2. In a preheated skillet or grill over medium heat, cook the salmon for 3-4 minutes per side until it flakes easily with a fork, and grill the asparagus alongside until tender.
3. Serve together, garnishing with a lemon wedge if desired. This simple, healthy meal offers protein and vegetables in minutes, perfect for a light lunch or dinner.

NUTRITIONAL VALUES (PER SERVING):

Calories: 250; Protein: 22g; Carbohydrates: 4g; Fiber: 2g; Total Fat: 16g

Caprese Salad

 Under 10 minutes

INGREDIENTS:

» 1 cup cherry tomatoes, halved
» ½ cup fresh mozzarella, cubed
» Fresh basil leaves, for garnish

INSTRUCTIONS:

1. In a mixing bowl, combine the halved cherry tomatoes and cubed mozzarella.
2. Add a few fresh basil leaves and drizzle with olive oil if desired.
3. Season lightly with salt and pepper, and toss gently. Serve immediately as a refreshing appetizer or side dish. This classic Italian salad is both simple and flavorful, showcasing the freshness of each ingredient.

NUTRITIONAL VALUES (PER SERVING):

Calories: 150; Protein: 8g; Carbohydrates: 5g; Fiber: 1g; Total Fat: 10g

Quick Beef Tacos

 Under 10 minutes

INGREDIENTS:

» ½ cup cooked ground beef
» 2 small corn tortillas
» 2 tablespoons shredded cheese

INSTRUCTIONS:

1. Warm the tortillas in a skillet for 1-2 minutes per side.
2. Divide the cooked ground beef between the tortillas and top with shredded cheese.
3. Garnish with salsa or a sprinkle of cilantro if desired. Serve immediately for a quick and delicious meal. These simple tacos are perfect for a light lunch or snack with a burst of Mexican flavor.

NUTRITIONAL VALUES (PER SERVING):

Calories: 200; Protein: 10g; Carbohydrates: 12g; Fiber: 2g; Total Fat: 12g

BLT Sandwich

 Under 10 minutes

INGREDIENTS:

» 2 slices toasted bread
» 2 slices cooked bacon
» 1 leaf lettuce, 1 slice tomato

INSTRUCTIONS:

1. Place the cooked bacon slices on one piece of toasted bread.
2. Add the lettuce leaf and tomato slice on top of the bacon.
3. Cover with the other piece of toasted bread, slice in half, and serve. This classic sandwich is easy to assemble and provides a satisfying combination of flavors and textures.

NUTRITIONAL VALUES (PER SERVING):

Calories: 300; Protein: 8g; Carbohydrates: 24g; Fiber: 2g; Total Fat: 18g

Chicken Quesadilla

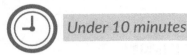 *Under 10 minutes*

INGREDIENTS:

» 1 flour tortilla
» ½ cup cooked chicken, shredded
» ¼ cup shredded cheese

INSTRUCTIONS:

1. Place the tortilla in a skillet over medium heat. Spread the shredded chicken and cheese evenly over one half of the tortilla.
2. Fold the tortilla in half, pressing down gently.
3. Cook for 2-3 minutes on each side until the tortilla is golden and the cheese is melted. Slice into wedges and serve warm. This quesadilla is a quick, tasty snack or light meal that's both filling and flavorful.

NUTRITIONAL VALUES (PER SERVING):

Calories: 250; Protein: 18g; Carbohydrates: 18g; Fiber: 1g; Total Fat: 12g

Greek Yogurt with Honey and Nuts

Under 10 minutes

INGREDIENTS:

» ½ cup Greek yogurt
» 1 tablespoon honey
» 1 tablespoon chopped nuts (almonds or walnuts)

INSTRUCTIONS:

1. In a bowl, spoon the Greek yogurt and drizzle with honey.
2. Add chopped nuts of your choice on top, to give it a extra crunch and taste.
3. Enjoy best if consumed right away as a wholesome serving of nutritionally balanced breakfast or snack. Featuring thick yogurt, the mild natural taste of honey, along with crunchy nutty bites this protein packed dish is tasty and healthy.

NUTRITIONAL VALUES (PER SERVING):

Calories: 180; Protein: 10g; Carbohydrates: 15g; Fiber: 1g; Total Fat: 8g

Tuna and Avocado Salad

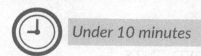 *Under 10 minutes*

INGREDIENTS:

» 1 can tuna in water, drained (5 oz)
» ½ avocado, diced
» 1 tablespoon lemon juice

INSTRUCTIONS:

1. In a bowl, combine the drained tuna and diced avocado.
2. Drizzle the lemon juice over the mixture and gently toss to combine.
3. Add salt and pepper to taste, and serve as a light meal or snack. This salad is creamy, protein-packed, and full of healthy fats, perfect for a quick lunch or dinner option.

NUTRITIONAL VALUES (PER SERVING):

Calories: 220; Protein: 20g; Carbohydrates: 5g; Fiber: 3g; Total Fat: 14g

Beef Stir-Fry with Bell Peppers

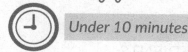 *Under 10 minutes*

INGREDIENTS:

» ½ cup thinly sliced beef
» 1 cup bell pepper strips (any color)
» 1 tablespoon soy sauce

INSTRUCTIONS:

1. In a skillet over medium-high heat, add the beef and stir-fry for 2-3 minutes until it begins to brown.
2. Add the bell peppers and soy sauce, stirring to coat everything evenly.
3. Cook for an additional 2-3 minutes until the peppers are tender-crisp. Serve warm, garnished with green onions if desired. This quick stir-fry is both flavorful and nutritious, ideal as a main dish.

NUTRITIONAL VALUES (PER SERVING):

Calories: 210; Protein: 18g; Carbohydrates: 6g; Fiber: 2g; Total Fat: 14g

Penne with Pesto

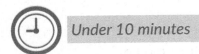 *Under 10 minutes*

INGREDIENTS:

» 1 cup cooked penne pasta
» 2 tablespoons pesto sauce
» 1 tablespoon grated Parmesan cheese

INSTRUCTIONS:

1. In a mixing bowl, toss the warm cooked penne with the pesto sauce until evenly coated.
2. Transfer to a serving dish and sprinkle with grated Parmesan.
3. Serve immediately for a quick, delicious meal with rich flavors. This pasta dish combines simplicity with taste, perfect for when you need something fast yet satisfying.

NUTRITIONAL VALUES (PER SERVING):

Calories: 300; Protein: 8g; Carbohydrates: 42g; Fiber: 2g; Total Fat: 12g

Mushroom and Cheese Omelette

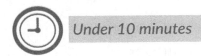 *Under 10 minutes*

INGREDIENTS:

» 2 large eggs, beaten
» ¼ cup mushrooms, sliced
» 2 tablespoons shredded cheese

INSTRUCTIONS:

1. In a skillet, on medium heat, add one or two tablespoons of butter: for 1-2 minutes or until the mushrooms are tender.
2. When the mushrooms are coated with oil pour the beaten eggs over the mushrooms and spread it across the pan.
3. Cover one half of the omelette in cheese, and let it cook for 2-3 minutes, after which it has been flipped. Serve hot. If you are in the lookout for some filling but very quick breakfast recipe, this savory omelette below will is perfect for you.

NUTRITIONAL VALUES (PER SERVING):

Calories: 200; Protein: 12g; Carbohydrates: 3g; Fiber: 1g; Total Fat: 16g

Chicken and Cucumber Salad

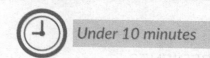 *Under 10 minutes*

INGREDIENTS:

» 1 cup cooked chicken breast, diced
» ½ cup cucumber, sliced
» 1 tablespoon Greek yogurt

INSTRUCTIONS:

1. In a bowl add diced chicken and sliced cucumber together.
2. Finally sprinkle Greek yogurt and gently turn the cooked vegetables over in order to distribute it evenly.
3. They should be seasoned with salt and pepper to taste, then taken immediately to the table. This light salad is the bomb, and you can have it anytime of the day, especially for lunch or a snack.

NUTRITIONAL VALUES (PER SERVING):

Calories: 150; Protein: 22g; Carbohydrates: 4g; Fiber: 1g; Total Fat: 5g

Chilled Tomato Soup (Gazpacho)

 Under 10 minutes

INGREDIENTS:

» 1 cup tomato juice
» ¼ cucumber, diced
» 1 tablespoon olive oil

INSTRUCTIONS:

1. Pour the tomato juice and chop cucumber into it and blend them.
2. Combine the olive oil into the mixture and blend till creamy.
3. Saute with salt and black pepper and then set aside to cool before being served. This is a delicious, low calorie soup that is excellent for hot weather and can make a lovely appetizer.

NUTRITIONAL VALUES (PER SERVING):

Calories: 100; Protein: 2g; Carbohydrates: 10g; Fiber: 2g; Total Fat: 7g

Sautéed Mushrooms with Garlic

 Under 10 minutes

INGREDIENTS:

- » 1 cup mushrooms, sliced
- » 1 tablespoon olive oil
- » 1 garlic clove, minced

INSTRUCTIONS:

1. Heat a skillet to medium and then cook olive oil and garlic before they turn brown.
2. Include mushrooms and cook this for 4-5 minutes until they are browned and soft.
3. In waiting, season with desired salt, pepper then serve warm. This healthy side dish only takes a few minutes to prepare and gives you that nice garlicky flavor.

NUTRITIONAL VALUES (PER SERVING):

Calories: 90; Protein: 2g; Carbohydrates: 6g; Fiber: 1g; Total Fat: 7g

Grilled Chicken Caesar Salad

 Under 10 minutes

INGREDIENTS:

- » 1 cup romaine lettuce, chopped
- » ½ cup cooked chicken breast, sliced
- » 1 tablespoon Caesar dressing

INSTRUCTIONS:

1. Take one bowl for raw romaine lettuce chopped and take other bowl for sliced chicken breast.
2. Pour over Caesar dressing, and toss gently.
3. Optional, this recipe can be garnished with Parmesan cheese or croutons, then it should be served immediately. This salad is ideal for everyone who would like to have a quick meal and get numerous exclusive and vivid tastes at lunch or dinner.

NUTRITIONAL VALUES (PER SERVING):

Calories: 220; Protein: 20g; Carbohydrates: 6g; Fiber: 2g; Total Fat: 12g

Veggie Pasta with Cream Sauce

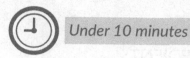 *Under 10 minutes*

INGREDIENTS:

» 1 cup cooked pasta
» ¼ cup heavy cream
» ¼ cup mixed vegetables (bell peppers, zucchini, etc.)

INSTRUCTIONS:

1. Heat the heavy cream using the skillet over medium heat.
2. Stir in the mixed vegetables and fry just long enough to cook them.
3. Add the cooked pasta to it and mix it in so that it blends with the other ingredients. It is hoped enjoyed straight away, as this dips best eaten as soon as it has been prepared, as this will provide the thick, rich texture.

NUTRITIONAL VALUES (PER SERVING):

Calories: 300; Protein: 8g; Carbohydrates: 40g; Fiber: 2g; Total Fat: 14g

Smoked Salmon on Whole Wheat Toast

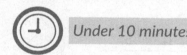 *Under 10 minutes*

INGREDIENTS:

» 1 slice whole wheat bread, toasted
» 2 oz smoked salmon
» 1 tablespoon cream cheese

INSTRUCTIONS:

1. Spread the cream cheese over the toasted bread.
2. Layer the smoked salmon on top, arranging evenly.
3. Garnish with fresh dill or capers if desired, and serve immediately. This simple toast offers a burst of flavor and healthy fats, ideal for a light breakfast or snack.

NUTRITIONAL VALUES (PER SERVING):

Calories: 180; Protein: 10g; Carbohydrates: 15g; Fiber: 3g; Total Fat: 8g

Spicy Lentil Soup

 Under 10 minutes

INGREDIENTS:

» 1 cup vegetable broth
» ¼ cup cooked lentils
» ½ teaspoon chili powder

INSTRUCTIONS:

1. In a saucepan over medium heat, add the vegetable broth and cooked lentils.
2. Stir in the chili powder, cooking until warmed through.
3. Serve hot, garnished with fresh herbs or a sprinkle of cayenne for added spice. This quick soup is hearty, protein-rich, and perfect for cool days.

NUTRITIONAL VALUES (PER SERVING):

Calories: 120; Protein: 6g; Carbohydrates: 15g; Fiber: 5g; Total Fat: 3g

Bacon and Egg Breakfast Bowl

 Under 10 minutes

INGREDIENTS:

» 2 strips cooked bacon, chopped
» 1 large egg, scrambled
» ¼ avocado, sliced

INSTRUCTIONS:

1. At this stage, spoon some of the scrambled egg on a bowl and add chopped bacon and avocado slices on top of the egg.
2. Add salt and pepper to serve a purpose of seasoning.
3. Perfect to be eaten fresh as a protein-packed breakfast food. This dish is easy to prepare, filling, and can be packed full of healthy ingredients to fill you up in the morning.

NUTRITIONAL VALUES (PER SERVING):

Calories: 250; Protein: 12g; Carbohydrates: 5g; Fiber: 3g; Total Fat: 20g

Shrimp Scampi

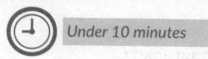

Under 10 minutes

INGREDIENTS:

» ½ cup shrimp, peeled and deveined
» 1 tablespoon butter
» 1 garlic clove, minced

INSTRUCTIONS:

1. In a skillet over medium heat, melt the butter and add minced garlic, cooking until fragrant.
2. Add shrimp, cooking for 2-3 minutes on each side until pink and cooked through.
3. Serve immediately, optionally garnished with parsley or a lemon wedge. This classic dish is flavorful and makes an elegant, quick meal.

NUTRITIONAL VALUES (PER SERVING):

Calories: 150; Protein: 14g; Carbohydrates: 1g; Fiber: 0g; Total Fat: 10g

Roasted Chickpeas with Lemon

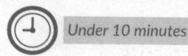

Under 10 minutes

INGREDIENTS:

» 1 cup canned chickpeas, drained
» 1 tablespoon olive oil
» Zest of ½ lemon

INSTRUCTIONS:

1. In a bowl, toss the chickpeas with olive oil and lemon zest.
2. Spread them on a baking sheet and roast in a preheated oven at 400°F for 8-10 minutes.
3. Serve as a crunchy, flavorful snack. These roasted chickpeas are rich in protein and fiber, perfect for a healthy munch.

NUTRITIONAL VALUES (PER SERVING):

Calories: 140; Protein: 6g; Carbohydrates: 20g; Fiber: 6g; Total Fat: 6g

Sautéed Kale with Garlic

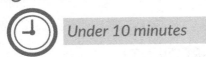 *Under 10 minutes*

INGREDIENTS:

» 1 cup kale, chopped
» 1 tablespoon olive oil
» 1 garlic clove, minced

INSTRUCTIONS:

1. In a skillet melt some olive oil and sauté the garlic until it becomes golden brown.
2. Kale should be added and s cooked for 4-5 minutes until it is soft.
3. Add salt and black pepper and then place in a warmer and wait then serve warm. Incredibly simple, but amazingly healthy, this side dish is sure to add great flavor to any dinner.

NUTRITIONAL VALUES (PER SERVING):

Calories: 80; Protein: 2g; Carbohydrates: 7g; Fiber: 2g; Total Fat: 6g

Avocado Smoothie

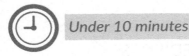 *Under 10 minutes*

INGREDIENTS:

» ½ avocado
» 1 cup milk (dairy or almond)
» 1 tablespoon honey

INSTRUCTIONS:

1. Avocado blended with milk and honey must be done in a blender.
2. Pulse until smooth and creamy and sweet enough depending on your liking to add more honey)
3. Drink forthwith it is one fabulous and nutrient containing beverage. I love this smoothie as it is heavy, nourishing with full fat and fibrous content.

NUTRITIONAL VALUES (PER SERVING):

Calories: 220; Protein: 4g; Carbohydrates: 20g; Fiber: 5g; Total Fat: 14g

Peanut Butter and Banana Toast

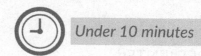 *Under 10 minutes*

INGREDIENTS:

» 1 slice whole-grain bread, toasted
» 1 tablespoon peanut butter
» ½ banana, sliced

INSTRUCTIONS:

1. Take the butter and spread it on each of the slices of bread, make sure that it is spread uniform all over.
2. Afterwards, layer the slices of banana over the peanut butter smiles.
3. Use as a quick meal to supplement it with honey where necessary. This toast compliments proteins and potassium thereby making this as a healthy toast.

NUTRITIONAL VALUES (PER SERVING):

Calories: 200; Protein: 6g; Carbohydrates: 28g; Fiber: 4g; Total Fat: 8g

Quinoa with Roasted Vegetables

Under 10 minutes

INGREDIENTS:

» ½ cup cooked quinoa
» ¼ cup roasted vegetables (bell peppers, zucchini, or carrots)
» 1 tablespoon olive oil

INSTRUCTIONS:

1. In a large bowl mix the cooked quinoa and the roasted vegetable together.
2. Pour on olive oil and turn the zabaglione to coat it well on the surface.
3. Don't should be to be served warm, as it can be a great side dish or even a light lunch. This flavoured quinoa is a source of fiber and plant protein; all the components of dieting as they make one feel fuller.

NUTRITIONAL VALUES (PER SERVING):

Calories: 180; Protein: 5g; Carbohydrates: 24g; Fiber: 3g; Total Fat: 7g

Pesto Chicken Wrap

 Under 10 minutes

INGREDIENTS:

» 1 whole wheat tortilla
» ½ cup cooked chicken breast, shredded
» 1 tablespoon pesto sauce

INSTRUCTIONS:

1. Spread the pesto sauce evenly over the tortilla.
2. Layer the shredded chicken on one side of the tortilla.
3. Roll up the tortilla tightly, slice in half, and serve. This wrap combines savory pesto with tender chicken for a quick, satisfying meal that's perfect for lunch or an on-the-go snack.

NUTRITIONAL VALUES (PER SERVING):

Calories: 250; Protein: 20g; Carbohydrates: 18g; Fiber: 3g; Total Fat: 12g

Tuna Melt

 Under 10 minutes

INGREDIENTS:

» 1 slice whole-grain bread
» ¼ cup canned tuna, drained
» 2 tablespoons shredded cheddar cheese

INSTRUCTIONS:

1. Place the bread slice on a baking sheet, top with tuna, and sprinkle with cheese.
2. Broil for 2-3 minutes until the cheese melts and the edges of the bread are golden.
3. Serve warm. This tuna melt is a quick, tasty option for lunch, delivering a warm, cheesy twist on classic tuna salad.

NUTRITIONAL VALUES (PER SERVING):

Calories: 220; Protein: 15g; Carbohydrates: 20g; Fiber: 3g; Total Fat: 10g

Carrot and Ginger Soup

 Under 10 minutes

INGREDIENTS:

- » 1 cup carrot juice
- » ½ teaspoon fresh ginger, grated
- » ¼ cup coconut milk

INSTRUCTIONS:

1. In a small pot over medium heat, combine carrot juice and grated ginger.
2. P.S The coconut milk should be added when the other ingredients are warm: stir for 5-7 minutes to heat.
3. salt and pepper respectively, and serve. This delicious soup is made from carrots and ginger and is very quick to make, so is ideal for a filling lunch.

NUTRITIONAL VALUES (PER SERVING):

Calories: 130; Protein: 1g; Carbohydrates: 15g; Fiber: 2g; Total Fat: 7g

Spinach and Ricotta Ravioli

 Under 10 minutes

INGREDIENTS:

- » 1 cup spinach and ricotta ravioli, cooked
- » 1 tablespoon olive oil
- » 1 tablespoon grated Parmesan

INSTRUCTIONS:

1. Drizzle the ravioli with olive oil and mix well until all the ravioli are coated with the olive oil.
2. Finally top with the remaining Parmesan cheese then serve. It may sound like a surprisingly traditional pasta dish, but it moist and filling with a great focus on the ricotta and spinach in the ravioli.

NUTRITIONAL VALUES (PER SERVING):

Calories: 280; Protein: 10g; Carbohydrates: 35g; Fiber: 2g; Total Fat: 10g

Turkey and Avocado Sandwich

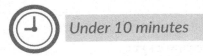 *Under 10 minutes*

INGREDIENTS:

» 2 slices whole-grain bread, toasted
» 2 oz sliced turkey breast
» ¼ avocado, sliced

INSTRUCTIONS:

1. Layer the turkey and avocado slices between the toasted bread slices.
2. Season with salt and pepper, and serve. This simple yet tasty sandwich is packed with lean protein and healthy fats, making it an ideal choice for a quick lunch.

NUTRITIONAL VALUES (PER SERVING):

Calories: 250; Protein: 15g; Carbohydrates: 28g; Fiber: 5g; Total Fat: 8g

Grilled Chicken and Veggie Skewers

 Under 10 minutes

INGREDIENTS:

» ½ cup cooked chicken breast, cubed
» ½ cup mixed bell peppers, cubed
» 1 tablespoon olive oil

INSTRUCTIONS:

1. Thread the chicken and bell peppers onto skewers, alternating pieces.
2. Brush with olive oil, and season with salt and pepper.
3. Grill for 2-3 minutes per side until warmed through. These skewers are colorful, nutritious, and ideal for a quick, flavorful meal.

NUTRITIONAL VALUES (PER SERVING):

Calories: 180; Protein: 18g; Carbohydrates: 5g; Fiber: 1g; Total Fat: 10g

Chickpea Salad

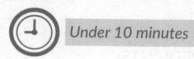 *Under 10 minutes*

INGREDIENTS:

» 1 cup canned chickpeas, drained
» ½ cup cherry tomatoes, halved
» 1 tablespoon lemon juice

INSTRUCTIONS:

1. In a bowl, combine chickpeas and cherry tomatoes.
2. Drizzle with lemon juice, tossing to coat evenly.
3. Season with salt and pepper, and serve. This salad is light, protein-rich, and filled with fresh, tangy flavors, perfect for a quick lunch or side dish.

NUTRITIONAL VALUES (PER SERVING):

Calories: 160; Protein: 6g; Carbohydrates: 24g; Fiber: 6g; Total Fat: 4g

Garlic Shrimp Pasta

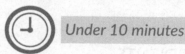 *Under 10 minutes*

INGREDIENTS:

» ½ cup cooked pasta
» ¼ cup shrimp, peeled and deveined
» 1 tablespoon olive oil

INSTRUCTIONS:

1. In a skillet over medium heat, add olive oil and shrimp, cooking for 2-3 minutes until shrimp is pink.
2. Add cooked pasta, tossing to coat in the oil.
3. Season with salt and pepper, and serve hot. This dish is packed with flavor, combining tender shrimp with pasta for a satisfying meal.

NUTRITIONAL VALUES (PER SERVING):

Calories: 250; Protein: 14g; Carbohydrates: 30g; Fiber: 2g; Total Fat: 8g

Tortilla Pizza

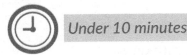 *Under 10 minutes*

INGREDIENTS:

- » 1 whole wheat tortilla
- » 2 tablespoons marinara sauce
- » ¼ cup shredded mozzarella cheese

INSTRUCTIONS:

1. Spread marinara sauce evenly over the tortilla, then sprinkle with shredded cheese.
2. Place on a baking sheet and broil for 3-4 minutes until cheese is melted and bubbly.
3. Serve warm, cut into slices. This quick tortilla pizza is a perfect snack or light meal, offering the classic pizza taste in minutes.

NUTRITIONAL VALUES (PER SERVING):

Calories: 220; Protein: 10g; Carbohydrates: 24g; Fiber: 3g; Total Fat: 10g

Veggie Soba Noodles

 Under 10 minutes

INGREDIENTS:

- » 1 cup cooked soba noodles
- » ½ cup mixed vegetables (bell peppers, carrots, snap peas)
- » 1 tablespoon soy sauce

INSTRUCTIONS:

1. In a skillet over medium heat, add the mixed vegetables and sauté until slightly tender.
2. Add the cooked soba noodles and soy sauce, tossing to coat.
3. Serve warm. This dish is quick, flavorful, and packed with veggies, making it a nutritious, light meal.

NUTRITIONAL VALUES (PER SERVING):

Calories: 180; Protein: 6g; Carbohydrates: 30g; Fiber: 3g; Total Fat: 4g

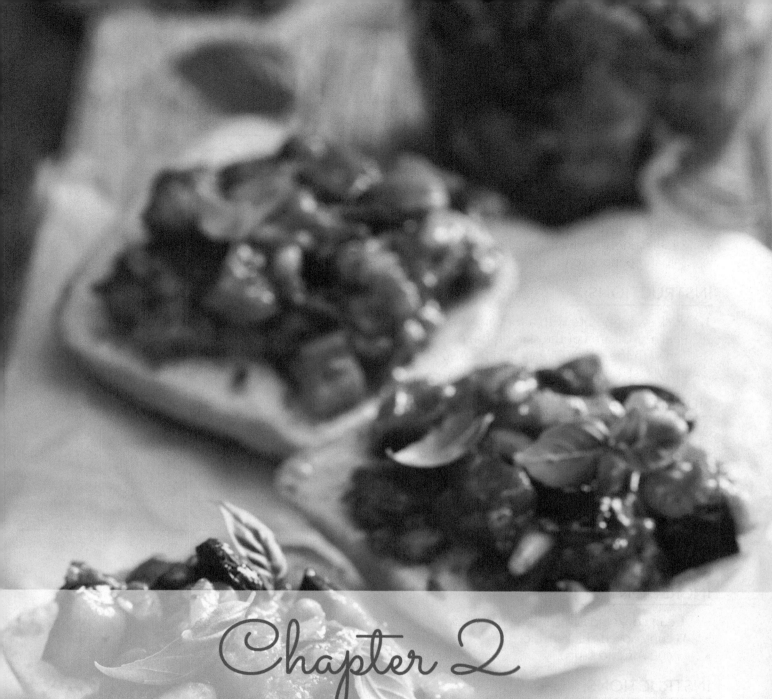

Chapter 2
15-MINUTE
Recipes

Quick meals ready in under 15 minutes.

Baked Sweet Potatoes with Sour Cream

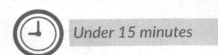 *Under 15 minutes*

INGREDIENTS:

» 1 medium sweet potato
» 2 tablespoons sour cream
» Salt and pepper to taste

INSTRUCTIONS:

1. Prick sweet potato with a fork and it's ready for microwaving on high for 5-7 minutes till soft.
2. Peel a small area of the skin on the potato and then use a fork to further loosen it up inside.
3. Top with the soured cream and then sprinkle the pepper and the salt on top of it. Can be eaten warm as a tasty, fast, healthy side dish or snack.

NUTRITIONAL VALUES (PER SERVING):

Calories: 150; Protein: 2g; Carbohydrates: 34g; Fiber: 5g; Total Fat: 2g

Chicken Alfredo Pasta

 Under 15 minutes

INGREDIENTS:

» 1 cup cooked pasta
» ½ cup cooked chicken, diced
» ¼ cup Alfredo sauce

INSTRUCTIONS:

1. In a saucepan over medium heat, combine the Alfredo sauce and diced chicken, stirring until warm.
2. Add the cooked pasta, tossing to coat with the sauce.
3. Serve hot, optionally garnished with Parmesan cheese. This creamy, comforting dish is ideal for a quick and satisfying meal.

NUTRITIONAL VALUES (PER SERVING):

Calories: 300; Protein: 18g; Carbohydrates: 35g; Fiber: 2g; Total Fat: 10g

Salmon Salad with Avocado

 Under 15 minutes

INGREDIENTS:

- » 3 oz cooked salmon, flaked
- » ½ avocado, diced
- » 1 tablespoon lemon juice

INSTRUCTIONS:

1. In a bowl, combine the flaked salmon and diced avocado.
2. Drizzle with lemon juice and gently toss to coat.
3. Season with salt and pepper to taste. This fresh, flavorful salad is packed with healthy fats and makes a light, satisfying meal or side dish.

NUTRITIONAL VALUES (PER SERVING):

Calories: 250; Protein: 15g; Carbohydrates: 8g; Fiber: 5g; Total Fat: 18g

Turkey Meatballs with Marinara

 Under 15 minutes

INGREDIENTS:

- » 4 pre-cooked turkey meatballs
- » ¼ cup marinara sauce
- » 1 tablespoon Parmesan cheese, grated

INSTRUCTIONS:

1. Place the meatballs and marinara sauce in a saucepan over medium heat, warming until heated through.
2. Top with grated Parmesan and serve. These quick meatballs are flavorful and perfect for a light meal or snack, offering a rich blend of Italian-inspired flavors in minutes.

NUTRITIONAL VALUES (PER SERVING):

Calories: 200; Protein: 15g; Carbohydrates: 8g; Fiber: 2g; Total Fat: 12g

Beef and Broccoli Stir-Fry

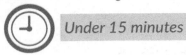 *Under 15 minutes*

INGREDIENTS:

- »   ½ cup thinly sliced beef
- »   1 cup broccoli florets
- »   1 tablespoon soy sauce

INSTRUCTIONS:

1. In a skillet over medium-high heat, add the beef slices, stirring until browned.
2. Add the broccoli and soy sauce, stirring to coat and cooking for 5 minutes or until broccoli is tender-crisp.
3. Serve warm. This classic stir-fry is quick, savory, and packed with protein and vegetables, perfect for a balanced meal in no time.

NUTRITIONAL VALUES (PER SERVING):

Calories: 220; Protein: 16g; Carbohydrates: 10g; Fiber: 3g; Total Fat: 12g

Bbq Chicken Sliders

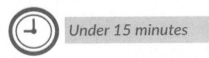 *Under 15 minutes*

INGREDIENTS:

- »   ½ cup cooked shredded chicken
- »   2 tablespoons BBQ sauce
- »   2 slider buns

INSTRUCTIONS:

1. In a small bowl, combine the shredded chicken with BBQ sauce, mixing until evenly coated.
2. Warm the mixture in a skillet over medium heat or microwave for 1-2 minutes.
3. Divide the BBQ chicken between the slider buns and serve immediately. These sliders are perfect for a quick, flavorful snack or appetizer, bringing a touch of smoky sweetness to each bite.

NUTRITIONAL VALUES (PER SERVING):

Calories: 250; Protein: 15g; Carbohydrates: 28g; Fiber: 2g; Total Fat: 8g

Shrimp Fajitas

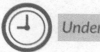 *Under 15 minutes*

INGREDIENTS:

» ½ cup shrimp, peeled and deveined
» ½ cup bell peppers, sliced
» 1 tablespoon fajita seasoning

INSTRUCTIONS:

1. In a skillet over medium-high heat, add the shrimp and bell peppers. Sprinkle with fajita seasoning and stir to coat.
2. Cook for 5-7 minutes until the shrimp is pink and cooked through, and peppers are tender.
3. Serve in tortillas or over rice. This quick, vibrant dish is packed with flavor and perfect for a speedy dinner with a hint of spice.

NUTRITIONAL VALUES (PER SERVING):

Calories: 180; Protein: 18g; Carbohydrates: 8g; Fiber: 2g; Total Fat: 6g

Grilled Eggplant with Mozzarella

 Under 15 minutes

INGREDIENTS:

» 1 small eggplant, sliced
» ¼ cup shredded mozzarella cheese
» 1 tablespoon olive oil

INSTRUCTIONS:

1. Brush the eggplant slices with olive oil and season with salt and pepper.
2. Grill the eggplant on medium heat for 3-4 minutes per side until tender.
3. Top each slice with mozzarella and grill until melted. This easy, cheesy appetizer is perfect for a quick bite, showcasing a smoky flavor with a creamy texture.

NUTRITIONAL VALUES (PER SERVING):

Calories: 160; Protein: 6g; Carbohydrates: 10g; Fiber: 4g; Total Fat: 12g

Caponata on Crostini

 Under 15 minutes

INGREDIENTS:

» ½ cup caponata (eggplant and tomato mixture)
» 4 slices baguette, toasted
» 1 tablespoon olive oil

INSTRUCTIONS:

1. Spread a thin layer of olive oil over the toasted baguette slices.
2. Spoon the caponata evenly over each slice, spreading gently.
3. Serve as a savory appetizer or light snack, offering a rich blend of Mediterranean flavors with each bite. This easy dish is bursting with the tangy taste of tomatoes, eggplant, and olives.

NUTRITIONAL VALUES (PER SERVING):

Calories: 140; Protein: 3g; Carbohydrates: 18g; Fiber: 2g; Total Fat: 7g

Tuna Pasta Salad

 Under 15 minutes

INGREDIENTS:

» 1 cup cooked pasta
» 1 can tuna, drained (5 oz)
» 2 tablespoons mayonnaise

INSTRUCTIONS:

1. In a large bowl, combine the pasta and tuna, flaking the tuna into bite-sized pieces.
2. Add mayonnaise and toss until the ingredients are evenly coated.
3. Season with salt and pepper and serve chilled or at room temperature. This pasta salad is light yet filling, perfect for a quick lunch or dinner with protein-packed flavor.

NUTRITIONAL VALUES (PER SERVING):

Calories: 300; Protein: 18g; Carbohydrates: 32g; Fiber: 2g; Total Fat: 12g

Spicy Ramen Noodles

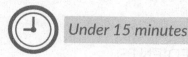 *Under 15 minutes*

INGREDIENTS:

- » 1 packet ramen noodles
- » 1 teaspoon chili paste
- » 1 tablespoon soy sauce

INSTRUCTIONS:

1. Cook ramen noodles according to package instructions, then drain.
2. In the pot, combine noodles with chili paste and soy sauce, stirring to coat evenly.
3. Serve hot, garnished with green onions or sesame seeds if desired. This quick dish brings a spicy twist to classic ramen, ideal for a flavorful meal in minutes.

NUTRITIONAL VALUES (PER SERVING):

Calories: 220; Protein: 5g; Carbohydrates: 30g; Fiber: 2g; Total Fat: 10g

Chicken Tenders with Honey Mustard

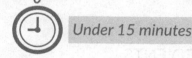 *Under 15 minutes*

INGREDIENTS:

- » ½ cup cooked chicken tenders
- » 1 tablespoon honey
- » 1 tablespoon Dijon mustard

INSTRUCTIONS:

1. In a small bowl, mix honey and Dijon mustard to make the dipping sauce.
2. Serve the chicken tenders warm with honey mustard on the side. This quick and easy dish is perfect for a snack or light meal with a touch of sweetness and tang.

NUTRITIONAL VALUES (PER SERVING):

Calories: 220; Protein: 18g; Carbohydrates: 10g; Fiber: 0g; Total Fat: 10g

Couscous with Vegetables

 Under 15 minutes

INGREDIENTS:

- » ½ cup couscous, cooked
- » ¼ cup mixed vegetables (bell peppers, carrots, peas)
- » 1 tablespoon olive oil

INSTRUCTIONS:

1. In a bowl, combine cooked couscous and mixed vegetables.
2. Drizzle with olive oil and toss gently.
3. Season with salt and pepper to taste, and serve warm or chilled. This quick, nutritious dish makes a light meal or side, full of flavor and healthy ingredients.

NUTRITIONAL VALUES (PER SERVING):

Calories: 200; Protein: 5g; Carbohydrates: 30g; Fiber: 4g; Total Fat: 8g

Tofu Stir-Fry

 Under 15 minutes

INGREDIENTS:

- » ½ cup tofu, cubed
- » ½ cup mixed vegetables (broccoli, bell pepper, carrots)
- » 1 tablespoon soy sauce

INSTRUCTIONS:

1. In a skillet over medium heat, add tofu and vegetables, stir-frying for 5-7 minutes until tender.
2. Drizzle with soy sauce, stirring to coat.
3. Serve warm. This quick, protein-rich stir-fry is packed with flavor and perfect for a light, balanced meal.

NUTRITIONAL VALUES (PER SERVING):

Calories: 180; Protein: 10g; Carbohydrates: 12g; Fiber: 3g; Total Fat: 10g

BLT Salad

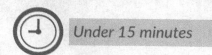 *Under 15 minutes*

INGREDIENTS:

» 2 cups lettuce, chopped
» 2 slices cooked bacon, chopped
» ½ cup cherry tomatoes, halved

INSTRUCTIONS:

1. In a large bowl, combine chopped lettuce, bacon, and cherry tomatoes.
2. Toss gently and serve immediately.
3. Optionally, drizzle with ranch or vinaigrette for extra flavor. This fresh salad captures the classic BLT flavors in a lighter, healthier form.

NUTRITIONAL VALUES (PER SERVING):

Calories: 140; Protein: 6g; Carbohydrates: 8g; Fiber: 3g; Total Fat: 10g

Roasted Tomato Soup

 Under 15 minutes

INGREDIENTS:

» 1 cup canned crushed tomatoes
» ¼ cup vegetable broth
» 1 teaspoon basil

INSTRUCTIONS:

1. In a saucepan, combine crushed tomatoes and vegetable broth, heating over medium heat until warm.
2. Stir in basil, seasoning with salt and pepper to taste.
3. Serve hot with a garnish of fresh basil if desired. This rich tomato soup is quick, comforting, and perfect for a chilly day.

NUTRITIONAL VALUES (PER SERVING):

Calories: 90; Protein: 2g; Carbohydrates: 15g; Fiber: 3g; Total Fat: 2g

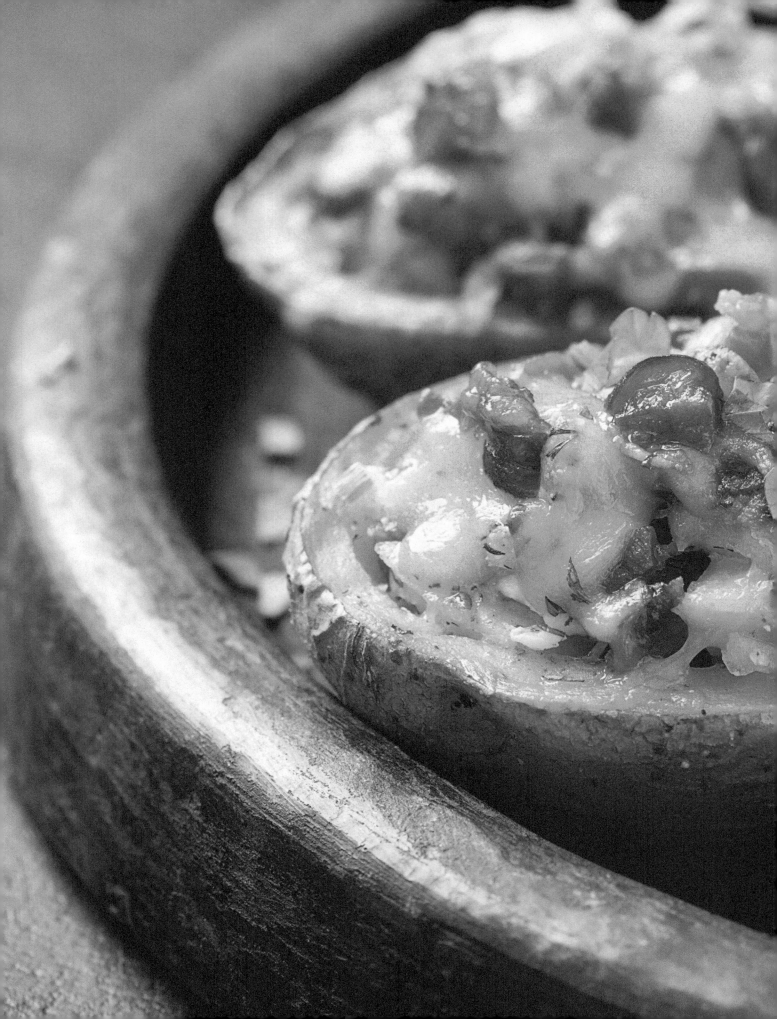

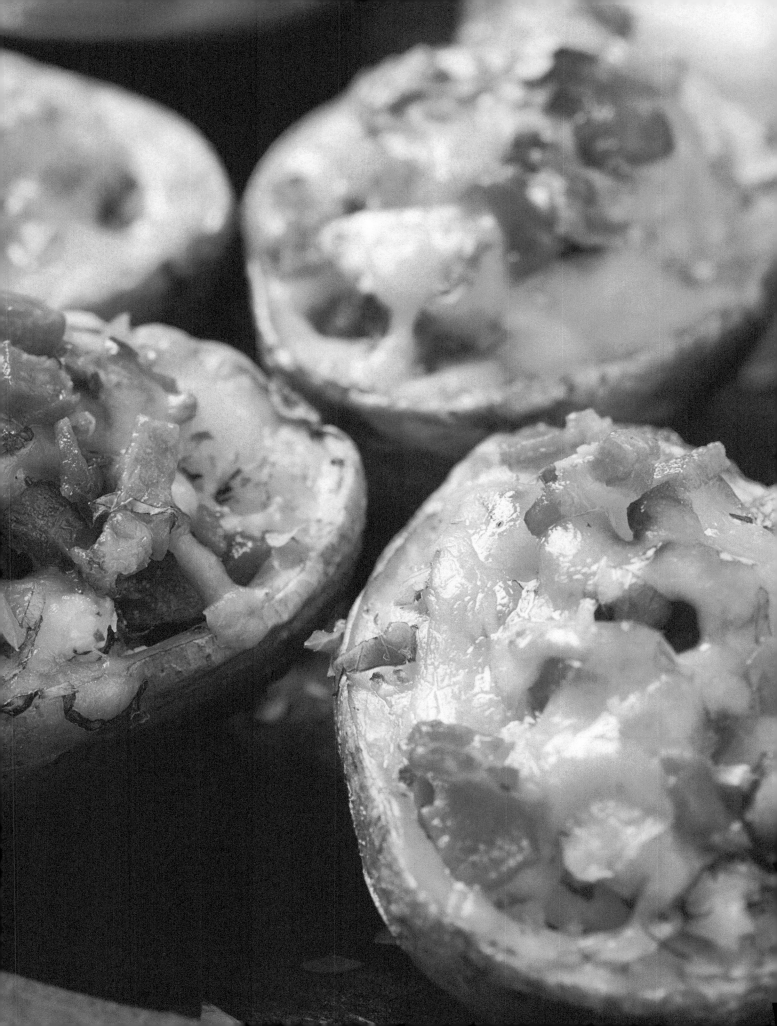

Grilled Fish Tacos

 Under 15 minutes

INGREDIENTS:

- » 2 small corn tortillas
- » ½ cup grilled fish, flaked
- » ¼ cup shredded cabbage

INSTRUCTIONS:

1. Place grilled fish on tortillas and top with shredded cabbage.
2. Squeeze fresh lime juice over the top, and serve immediately. These tacos are light, flavorful, and perfect for a quick, healthy meal.

NUTRITIONAL VALUES (PER SERVING):

Calories: 180; Protein: 15g; Carbohydrates: 18g; Fiber: 3g; Total Fat: 6g

Quinoa and Kale Bowl

 Under 15 minutes

INGREDIENTS:

- » ½ cup cooked quinoa
- » ½ cup chopped kale
- » 1 tablespoon olive oil

INSTRUCTIONS:

1. In a bowl, combine the quinoa and kale, drizzling with olive oil.
2. Toss gently and season with salt and pepper.
3. Serve as a light meal or side. This bowl is nutrient-dense, with protein and greens for a quick, wholesome option.

NUTRITIONAL VALUES (PER SERVING):

Calories: 160; Protein: 5g; Carbohydrates: 22g; Fiber: 4g; Total Fat: 6g

Quick Beef Chili

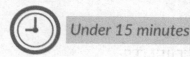 *Under 15 minutes*

INGREDIENTS:

» ½ cup ground beef, cooked
» ½ cup canned kidney beans
» ¼ cup tomato sauce

INSTRUCTIONS:

1. In a saucepan, combine cooked ground beef, kidney beans, and tomato sauce, stirring well.
2. Heat over medium heat until warm.
3. Season with chili powder if desired, and serve hot. This quick chili is hearty and perfect for a fast, comforting meal.

NUTRITIONAL VALUES (PER SERVING):

Calories: 220; Protein: 14g; Carbohydrates: 18g; Fiber: 4g; Total Fat: 10g

Grilled Portobello Mushrooms

 Under 15 minutes

INGREDIENTS:

» 2 portobello mushrooms
» 1 tablespoon balsamic vinegar
» 1 tablespoon olive oil

INSTRUCTIONS:

1. Brush mushrooms with balsamic vinegar and olive oil.
2. Grill over medium heat for 5-7 minutes until tender.
3. Serve warm as a side or add to a salad for a savory, meat-free option. Grilled portobellos bring a rich, umami flavor, making them a perfect addition to any meal.

NUTRITIONAL VALUES (PER SERVING):

Calories: 100; Protein: 2g; Carbohydrates: 6g; Fiber: 2g; Total Fat: 8g

Fried Polenta with Cheese

 Under 15 minutes

INGREDIENTS:

»   1 cup pre-cooked polenta, sliced
»   ¼ cup shredded mozzarella cheese
»   1 tablespoon olive oil

INSTRUCTIONS:

1.   In a skillet over medium heat, warm the olive oil. Add polenta slices, frying for 3-4 minutes per side until golden and crispy.
2.   Sprinkle mozzarella cheese over the polenta slices, covering until melted.
3.   Serve warm as a savory snack or side dish. The crispy polenta with melted cheese offers a comforting, flavorful bite that's quick to prepare.

NUTRITIONAL VALUES (PER SERVING):

Calories: 180; Protein: 6g; Carbohydrates: 15g; Fiber: 2g; Total Fat: 10g

Cauliflower Rice with Herbs

 Under 15 minutes

INGREDIENTS:

»   1 cup cauliflower rice
»   1 tablespoon olive oil
»   1 tablespoon chopped fresh herbs (parsley, basil)

INSTRUCTIONS:

1.   In a skillet over medium heat, warm olive oil and add cauliflower rice.
2.   Sauté for 5 minutes until tender, stirring occasionally.
3.   Add fresh herbs and season with salt and pepper. Serve warm. This light, herbaceous cauliflower rice is a healthy, low-carb alternative to traditional rice.

NUTRITIONAL VALUES (PER SERVING):

Calories: 80; Protein: 2g; Carbohydrates: 5g; Fiber: 2g; Total Fat: 6g

Spinach and Feta Stuffed Peppers

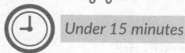 **Under 15 minutes**

INGREDIENTS:

» 1 bell pepper, halved and seeded
» ½ cup fresh spinach, chopped
» ¼ cup crumbled feta cheese

INSTRUCTIONS:

1. In a bowl, mix spinach and feta cheese. Stuff the mixture into each half of the bell pepper.
2. Microwave for 2-3 minutes or bake at 375°F for 10 minutes until peppers are tender.
3. Serve warm. This easy recipe combines creamy feta and fresh spinach in a vibrant pepper shell, perfect as a light meal.

NUTRITIONAL VALUES (PER SERVING):

Calories: 120; Protein: 4g; Carbohydrates: 8g; Fiber: 3g; Total Fat: 8g

Tomato Basil Bruschetta

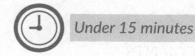 **Under 15 minutes**

INGREDIENTS:

» 4 slices baguette, toasted
» 1 cup diced tomatoes
» 1 tablespoon chopped fresh basil

INSTRUCTIONS:

1. In a bowl, mix diced tomatoes and basil, seasoning with salt and pepper.
2. Spoon the tomato mixture onto the toasted baguette slices.
3. Serve immediately as a refreshing appetizer. This bruschetta offers a fresh, vibrant taste with juicy tomatoes and aromatic basil on crisp bread.

NUTRITIONAL VALUES (PER SERVING):

Calories: 130; Protein: 3g; Carbohydrates: 20g; Fiber: 1g; Total Fat: 4g

Shrimp and Couscous Salad

 Under 15 minutes

INGREDIENTS:

» ½ cup cooked couscous
» ¼ cup cooked shrimp
» 1 tablespoon lemon juice

INSTRUCTIONS:

1. In a bowl, combine the couscous and shrimp.
2. Drizzle with lemon juice, tossing to coat.
3. Serve chilled or at room temperature, seasoned with salt and pepper. This light, zesty salad is perfect for a quick, healthy meal, with tender shrimp and fluffy couscous.

NUTRITIONAL VALUES (PER SERVING):

Calories: 150; Protein: 10g; Carbohydrates: 20g; Fiber: 2g; Total Fat: 4g

Bacon-Wrapped Asparagus

 Under 15 minutes

INGREDIENTS:

» 4 asparagus spears
» 2 slices bacon

INSTRUCTIONS:

1. Wrap each bacon slice around two asparagus spears.
2. Place in a skillet over medium heat and cook for 5-7 minutes, turning until bacon is crispy.
3. Serve warm as an appetizer or side. This simple, savory dish combines crispy bacon with tender asparagus for a satisfying bite.

NUTRITIONAL VALUES (PER SERVING):

Calories: 120; Protein: 5g; Carbohydrates: 2g; Fiber: 1g; Total Fat: 10g

Pasta Carbonara

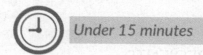 *Under 15 minutes*

INGREDIENTS:

» 1 cup cooked pasta
» 1 egg, beaten
» 2 tablespoons grated Parmesan

INSTRUCTIONS:

1. In a skillet with the pasta over low heat, add the beaten egg, stirring until it coats the pasta.
2. Sprinkle with Parmesan and toss to combine.
3. Serve warm, seasoned with black pepper. This creamy, cheesy dish is a quick Italian favorite.

NUTRITIONAL VALUES (PER SERVING):

Calories: 300; Protein: 12g; Carbohydrates: 42g; Fiber: 2g; Total Fat: 8g

Baked Zucchini Boats

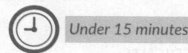 *Under 15 minutes*

INGREDIENTS:

» 1 zucchini, halved and hollowed
» ¼ cup marinara sauce
» 2 tablespoons shredded mozzarella

INSTRUCTIONS:

1. Fill zucchini halves with marinara sauce and sprinkle with mozzarella.
2. Bake at 400°F for 10 minutes until cheese is melted.
3. Serve warm as a tasty, veggie-packed side. This baked zucchini boat is a fun, flavorful way to enjoy vegetables with a cheesy touch.

NUTRITIONAL VALUES (PER SERVING):

Calories: 100; Protein: 5g; Carbohydrates: 6g; Fiber: 2g; Total Fat: 6g

Bbq Chicken Quesadillas

 Under 15 minutes

INGREDIENTS:

» 1 flour tortilla
» ¼ cup cooked chicken, shredded
» 1 tablespoon BBQ sauce

INSTRUCTIONS:

1. Spread BBQ sauce over the tortilla, then sprinkle with chicken.
2. Fold in half and cook in a skillet over medium heat for 2-3 minutes per side until crispy.
3. Serve hot, cut into wedges. This quesadilla is a quick, savory snack with smoky BBQ flavor.

NUTRITIONAL VALUES (PER SERVING):

Calories: 220; Protein: 12g; Carbohydrates: 20g; Fiber: 2g; Total Fat: 10g

Chicken Stir-Fry with Vegetables

 Under 15 minutes

INGREDIENTS:

» ½ cup cooked chicken, sliced
» ½ cup mixed vegetables (carrots, bell peppers, snap peas)
» 1 tablespoon soy sauce

INSTRUCTIONS:

1. In a skillet, stir-fry chicken and vegetables over medium heat for 5 minutes.
2. Add soy sauce and toss to coat.
3. Serve immediately. This stir-fry is a nutritious, colorful dish with a balance of protein and veggies.

NUTRITIONAL VALUES (PER SERVING):

Calories: 180; Protein: 14g; Carbohydrates: 10g; Fiber: 3g; Total Fat: 8g

Soba Noodles with Peanut Sauce

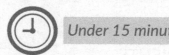 *Under 15 minutes*

INGREDIENTS:

- » 1 cup cooked soba noodles
- » 1 tablespoon peanut butter
- » 1 tablespoon soy sauce

INSTRUCTIONS:

1. In a bowl, mix peanut butter and soy sauce, then toss with cooked noodles.
2. Serve warm or chilled, garnished with green onions if desired. This dish has a creamy, nutty flavor and is a quick, satisfying meal.

NUTRITIONAL VALUES (PER SERVING):

Calories: 250; Protein: 8g; Carbohydrates: 35g; Fiber: 3g; Total Fat: 10g

Garlic Butter Shrimp

 Under 15 minutes

INGREDIENTS:

- » ½ cup shrimp, peeled and deveined
- » 1 tablespoon butter
- » 1 garlic clove, minced

INSTRUCTIONS:

1. In a skillet, melt butter and add garlic, cooking until fragrant.
2. Add shrimp and cook for 2-3 minutes per side until pink.
3. Serve hot with a garnish of parsley if desired. This dish is rich, flavorful, and perfect as an appetizer or main course.

NUTRITIONAL VALUES (PER SERVING):

Calories: 160; Protein: 12g; Carbohydrates: 1g; Fiber: 0g; Total Fat: 12g

Roasted Cauliflower with Parmesan

 Under 15 minutes

INGREDIENTS:

» 1 cup cauliflower florets
» 1 tablespoon olive oil
» 2 tablespoons grated Parmesan

INSTRUCTIONS:

1. Toss cauliflower with olive oil and Parmesan, then spread on a baking sheet.
2. Roast at 400°F for 10-12 minutes until golden.
3. Serve as a delicious side, crispy and full of flavor. Roasted cauliflower with Parmesan adds a savory, cheesy twist to the vegetable.

NUTRITIONAL VALUES (PER SERVING):

Calories: 110; Protein: 4g; Carbohydrates: 6g; Fiber: 3g; Total Fat: 8g

Pita with Hummus and Veggies

 Under 15 minutes

INGREDIENTS:

» 1 whole wheat pita, halved
» 2 tablespoons hummus
» ¼ cup mixed veggies (cucumber, bell pepper, carrot)

INSTRUCTIONS:

1. Spread hummus inside the pita halves.
2. Fill with mixed veggies, pressing gently.
3. Serve immediately. This simple, nutritious snack is a refreshing mix of creamy hummus and crunchy vegetables.

NUTRITIONAL VALUES (PER SERVING):

Calories: 150; Protein: 5g; Carbohydrates: 20g; Fiber: 4g; Total Fat: 5g

Creamy Avocado Pasta

 Under 15 minutes

INGREDIENTS:

» 1 cup cooked pasta
» ½ avocado, mashed
» 1 tablespoon lemon juice

INSTRUCTIONS:

1. In a bowl, combine mashed avocado and lemon juice, then toss with pasta.
2. Serve warm or chilled, seasoned with salt and pepper. This creamy, plant-based pasta dish is both rich and refreshing, ideal for a light meal.

NUTRITIONAL VALUES (PER SERVING):

Calories: 280; Protein: 6g; Carbohydrates: 42g; Fiber: 6g; Total Fat: 10g

Spinach and Cheese Quesadilla

 Under 15 minutes

INGREDIENTS:

» 1 flour tortilla
» ½ cup spinach, chopped
» ¼ cup shredded cheese

INSTRUCTIONS:

1. Layer spinach and cheese on one side of the tortilla. Fold in half.
2. Cook in a skillet over medium heat for 3-4 minutes on each side.
3. Serve warm, cut into wedges. This quesadilla offers a quick, nutritious option with melted cheese and fresh spinach.

NUTRITIONAL VALUES (PER SERVING):

Calories: 200; Protein: 8g; Carbohydrates: 20g; Fiber: 3g; Total Fat: 10g

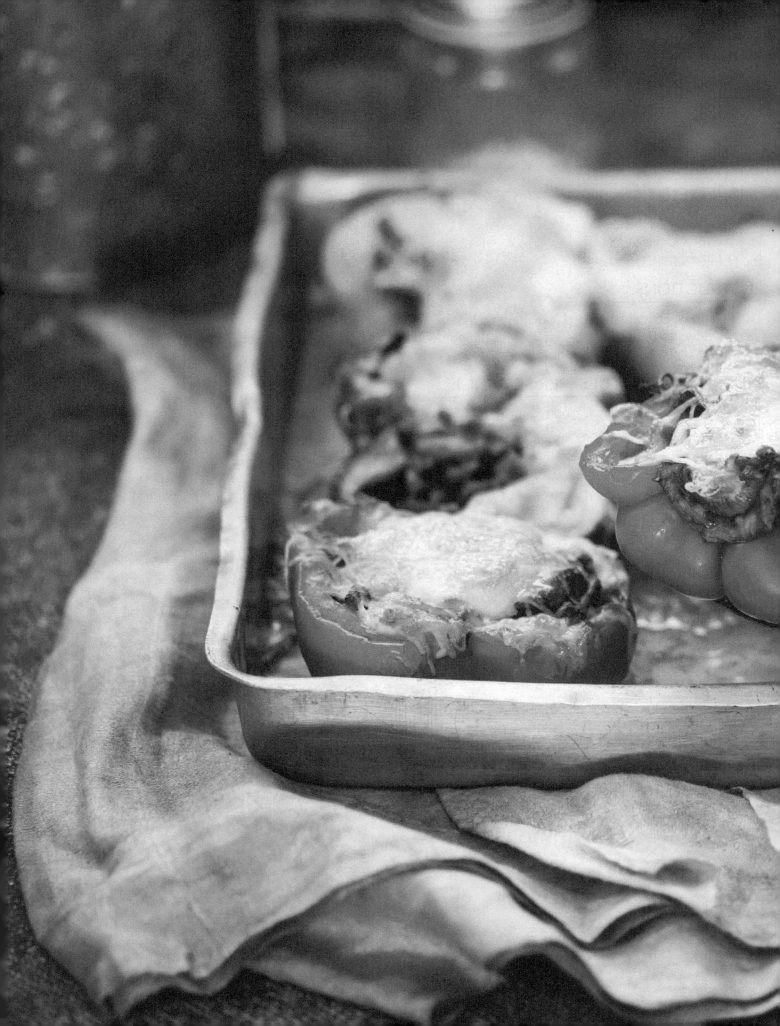

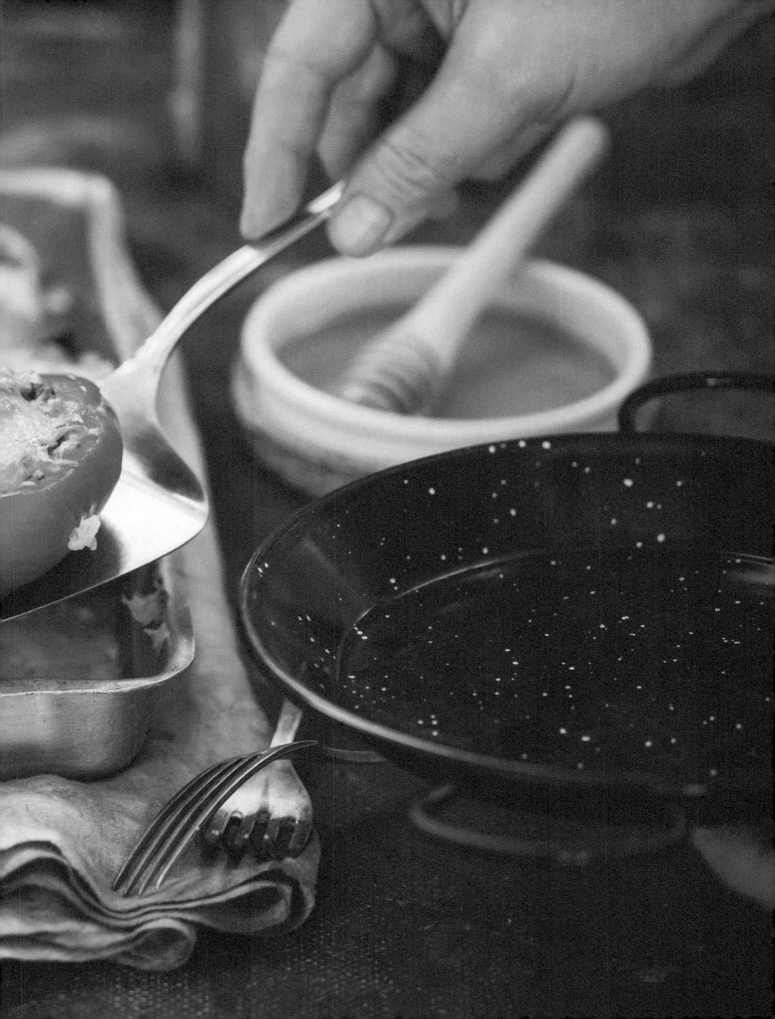

Veggie Frittata

 Under 15 minutes

INGREDIENTS:

» 2 large eggs, beaten
» ¼ cup mixed vegetables (bell peppers, spinach, onions)
» 1 tablespoon olive oil

INSTRUCTIONS:

1. In a skillet over medium heat, warm the olive oil and add mixed vegetables. Sauté until tender.
2. Pour the beaten eggs over the vegetables, spreading evenly.
3. Cook for 3-4 minutes until the eggs are set, then fold or serve as-is. This quick veggie frittata is perfect for a protein-packed breakfast or light meal, featuring vibrant vegetables and fluffy eggs.

NUTRITIONAL VALUES (PER SERVING):

Calories: 180; Protein: 10g; Carbohydrates: 5g; Fiber: 2g; Total Fat: 14g

Shrimp Salad with Lemon Dressing

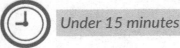 *Under 15 minutes*

INGREDIENTS:

» ½ cup cooked shrimp
» 1 cup mixed greens
» 1 tablespoon lemon juice

INSTRUCTIONS:

1. In a bowl, combine cooked shrimp and mixed greens.
2. Drizzle with lemon juice, and toss gently to coat.
3. Season with salt and pepper, and serve immediately. This refreshing salad brings together tender shrimp with crisp greens and a tangy lemon dressing, ideal for a light and healthy meal.

NUTRITIONAL VALUES (PER SERVING):

Calories: 120; Protein: 10g; Carbohydrates: 5g; Fiber: 1g; Total Fat: 7g

Lentil and Carrot Soup

 Under 15 minutes

INGREDIENTS:

» 1 cup vegetable broth
» ¼ cup cooked lentils
» ¼ cup carrots, diced

INSTRUCTIONS:

1. In a saucepan, combine vegetable broth, lentils, and carrots.
2. Heat over medium heat for 5-7 minutes until warm and carrots are tender.
3. Serve hot, seasoned with salt and pepper. This quick soup is nourishing, flavorful, and perfect for a comforting, protein-rich meal.

NUTRITIONAL VALUES (PER SERVING):

Calories: 100; Protein: 6g; Carbohydrates: 15g; Fiber: 4g; Total Fat: 2g

Grilled Cheese with Tomato Soup

 Under 15 minutes

INGREDIENTS:

» 2 slices bread
» 2 slices cheddar cheese
» 1 cup tomato soup (store-bought or homemade)

INSTRUCTIONS:

1. Place cheese between bread slices and cook in a skillet until golden and melted, about 2-3 minutes per side.
2. Heat tomato soup in a saucepan until warm.
3. Serve grilled cheese with soup for dipping. This classic pairing is comforting and quick, ideal for a cozy meal.

NUTRITIONAL VALUES (PER SERVING):

Calories: 300; Protein: 10g; Carbohydrates: 35g; Fiber: 2g; Total Fat: 14g

Chicken with Spinach and Mushrooms

 Under 15 minutes

INGREDIENTS:

- » ½ cup cooked chicken breast, sliced
- » ½ cup fresh spinach
- » ¼ cup mushrooms, sliced

INSTRUCTIONS:

1. In a skillet, sauté mushrooms over medium heat until softened, then add spinach.
2. Add the cooked chicken, stirring until everything is warmed through.
3. Serve immediately. This dish combines tender chicken, earthy mushrooms, and fresh spinach for a balanced and flavorful meal.

NUTRITIONAL VALUES (PER SERVING):

Calories: 180; Protein: 20g; Carbohydrates: 4g; Fiber: 2g; Total Fat: 8g

Vegan Buddha Bowl

 Under 15 minutes

INGREDIENTS:

- » ½ cup cooked quinoa
- » ¼ cup chickpeas
- » ¼ cup diced cucumber

INSTRUCTIONS:

1. In a bowl, layer the cooked quinoa, chickpeas, and cucumber.
2. Drizzle with olive oil and season with salt and pepper.
3. Serve as a nutritious, plant-based meal, packed with protein and fiber. This vegan Buddha bowl offers a fresh, satisfying mix of flavors and textures.

NUTRITIONAL VALUES (PER SERVING):

Calories: 220; Protein: 8g; Carbohydrates: 32g; Fiber: 6g; Total Fat: 7g

Penne with Ricotta and Spinach

 Under 15 minutes

INGREDIENTS:

» 1 cup cooked penne pasta
» ¼ cup ricotta cheese
» ½ cup fresh spinach

INSTRUCTIONS:

1. Toss the warm pasta with ricotta cheese until evenly coated.
2. Add spinach, stirring until wilted.
3. Serve immediately. This creamy, comforting pasta dish combines soft ricotta and fresh spinach for a balanced, satisfying meal.

NUTRITIONAL VALUES (PER SERVING):

Calories: 280; Protein: 10g; Carbohydrates: 42g; Fiber: 3g; Total Fat: 8g

Pork Tenderloin with Apples

 Under 15 minutes

INGREDIENTS:

» ½ cup cooked pork tenderloin, sliced
» ½ apple, thinly sliced
» 1 tablespoon olive oil

INSTRUCTIONS:

1. In a skillet over medium heat, warm olive oil and add apple slices, cooking until tender.
2. Add pork tenderloin, stirring until warmed through.
3. Serve immediately, combining savory pork with sweet apple flavors. This dish is both hearty and balanced, perfect for a quick, elegant meal.

NUTRITIONAL VALUES (PER SERVING):

Calories: 220; Protein: 18g; Carbohydrates: 10g; Fiber: 2g; Total Fat: 12g

Grilled Shrimp with Mango Salsa

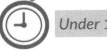 *Under 15 minutes*

INGREDIENTS:

» ½ cup shrimp, peeled and deveined
» ¼ cup diced mango
» 1 tablespoon chopped cilantro

INSTRUCTIONS:

1. Grill the shrimp over medium heat for 2-3 minutes per side until pink and cooked through.
2. In a bowl, combine diced mango and cilantro.
3. Serve the shrimp with mango salsa on top. This fresh and tropical dish pairs sweet mango with savory grilled shrimp, ideal for a quick and refreshing meal.

NUTRITIONAL VALUES (PER SERVING):

Calories: 150; Protein: 12g; Carbohydrates: 10g; Fiber: 1g; Total Fat: 6g

Kale Caesar Salad

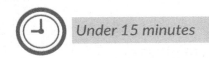 *Under 15 minutes*

INGREDIENTS:

» 2 cups kale, chopped
» 2 tablespoons Caesar dressing
» 1 tablespoon grated Parmesan cheese

INSTRUCTIONS:

1. In a large bowl, massage the chopped kale with Caesar dressing for 1-2 minutes until softened.
2. Add grated Parmesan cheese and toss to coat.
3. Serve immediately, optionally topped with croutons for extra crunch. This quick kale Caesar salad is a healthy twist on the classic, featuring nutrient-dense kale with creamy dressing and savory Parmesan. Perfect as a side dish or light meal.

NUTRITIONAL VALUES (PER SERVING):

Calories: 140; Protein: 5g; Carbohydrates: 8g; Fiber: 3g; Total Fat: 10g

Bbq Chicken Pizza

 Under 15 minutes

INGREDIENTS:

- » 1 small pre-baked pizza crust
- » ¼ cup cooked chicken, shredded
- » 2 tablespoons BBQ sauce
- » ¼ cup shredded mozzarella cheese

INSTRUCTIONS:

1. Spread BBQ sauce over the pizza crust, then layer with shredded chicken and mozzarella.
2. Bake in a preheated oven at 400°F for 8-10 minutes until cheese is melted and bubbly.
3. Slice and serve warm. This BBQ chicken pizza is a flavorful, quick meal with smoky BBQ sauce, tender chicken, and melty cheese. Perfect for a satisfying dinner or snack.

NUTRITIONAL VALUES (PER SERVING):

Calories: 280; Protein: 12g; Carbohydrates: 30g; Fiber: 2g; Total Fat: 12g

Roasted Brussels Sprouts with Bacon

 Under 15 minutes

INGREDIENTS:

- » 1 cup Brussels sprouts, halved
- » 2 slices bacon, chopped
- » Salt and pepper to taste

INSTRUCTIONS:

1. In a skillet over medium heat, cook chopped bacon until crispy. Remove and set aside, leaving a small amount of fat in the skillet.
2. Add Brussels sprouts, cut side down, and cook for 5-7 minutes until golden and tender.
3. Mix in bacon pieces, season with salt and pepper, and serve warm. This savory dish combines crispy bacon with caramelized Brussels sprouts for a delicious side.

NUTRITIONAL VALUES (PER SERVING):

Calories: 160; Protein: 6g; Carbohydrates: 8g; Fiber: 3g; Total Fat: 12g

Baked Chicken Wings

 Under 15 minutes

INGREDIENTS:

» 6 chicken wings
» 1 tablespoon olive oil
» Salt, pepper, and paprika to taste

INSTRUCTIONS:

1. Preheat the oven to 425°F. Toss chicken wings with olive oil, salt, pepper, and paprika.
2. Arrange on a baking sheet and bake for 10-12 minutes until crispy and golden.
3. Serve hot with your favorite dipping sauce. These baked wings are flavorful and crispy, perfect as a quick appetizer or main dish.

NUTRITIONAL VALUES (PER SERVING):

Calories: 220; Protein: 15g; Carbohydrates: 1g; Fiber: 0g; Total Fat: 16g

Grilled Cheese with Avocado

 Under 15 minutes

INGREDIENTS:

» 2 slices whole-grain bread
» 2 slices cheddar cheese
» ½ avocado, sliced

INSTRUCTIONS:

1. Layer cheddar cheese and avocado slices between the bread slices.
2. Grill in a skillet over medium heat for 3-4 minutes on each side until golden and cheese is melted.
3. Serve warm. This twist on the classic grilled cheese adds creamy avocado for extra richness and nutrition, making it an irresistible comfort food.

NUTRITIONAL VALUES (PER SERVING):

Calories: 300; Protein: 10g; Carbohydrates: 32g; Fiber: 5g; Total Fat: 18g

Seared Tuna with Sesame Seeds

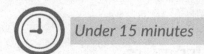 *Under 15 minutes*

INGREDIENTS:

» 1 tuna steak (about 4 oz)
» 1 tablespoon sesame seeds
» 1 tablespoon olive oil

INSTRUCTIONS:

1. Coat the tuna steak with sesame seeds on both sides.
2. In a skillet over medium-high heat, warm olive oil, and sear the tuna for 1-2 minutes on each side until golden but still rare inside.
3. Serve immediately, optionally garnished with soy sauce or wasabi. This quick, protein-rich dish has a nutty, savory flavor and is perfect for a light, healthy meal.

NUTRITIONAL VALUES (PER SERVING):

Calories: 200; Protein: 25g; Carbohydrates: 1g; Fiber: 0g; Total Fat: 10g

Greek Salad with Chicken

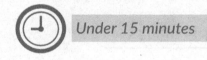 *Under 15 minutes*

INGREDIENTS:

» 1 cup romaine lettuce, chopped
» ½ cup cooked chicken breast, diced
» ¼ cup cucumber, sliced
» 2 tablespoons feta cheese, crumbled

INSTRUCTIONS:

1. In a bowl, combine lettuce, chicken, cucumber, and feta cheese.
2. Toss with olive oil and a squeeze of lemon juice, then season with salt and pepper.
3. Serve immediately. This Greek salad with chicken is refreshing, packed with protein, and full of Mediterranean flavors, perfect for a quick and healthy meal.

NUTRITIONAL VALUES (PER SERVING):

Calories: 220; Protein: 20g; Carbohydrates: 8g; Fiber: 2g; Total Fat: 12g

Steak Fajitas

 Under 15 minutes

INGREDIENTS:

» ½ cup thinly sliced steak
» ½ cup bell pepper strips
» 1 tablespoon fajita seasoning

INSTRUCTIONS:

1. In a skillet over medium-high heat, add steak and bell peppers, sprinkling with fajita seasoning.
2. Sauté for 5-7 minutes until steak is cooked to your liking and peppers are tender.
3. Serve in warm tortillas. These quick fajitas offer a smoky, flavorful meal with tender steak and vibrant peppers.

NUTRITIONAL VALUES (PER SERVING):

Calories: 250; Protein: 20g; Carbohydrates: 6g; Fiber: 2g; Total Fat: 16g

Grilled Corn on the Cob

 Under 15 minutes

INGREDIENTS:

» 2 ears of corn, husked
» 1 tablespoon butter, melted
» Salt and pepper to taste

INSTRUCTIONS:

1. Brush each ear of corn with melted butter and season with salt and pepper.
2. Grill over medium heat for 5-7 minutes, rotating occasionally, until slightly charred.
3. Serve hot. Grilled corn on the cob is sweet, smoky, and full of flavor, making it a perfect side for any summer meal.

NUTRITIONAL VALUES (PER SERVING):

Calories: 120; Protein: 3g; Carbohydrates: 20g; Fiber: 2g; Total Fat: 4g

Stuffed Bell Peppers

 Under 15 minutes

INGREDIENTS:

» 1 bell pepper, halved and seeded
» ½ cup cooked rice
» ¼ cup ground beef, cooked

INSTRUCTIONS:

1. In a bowl, mix the rice and ground beef, seasoning with salt and pepper.
2. Fill each bell pepper half with the rice and beef mixture.
3. Microwave or bake at 375°F for 10 minutes until the pepper is tender. This dish combines hearty rice and beef with the fresh crunch of bell pepper for a quick, nutritious meal.

NUTRITIONAL VALUES (PER SERVING):

Calories: 180; Protein: 8g; Carbohydrates: 22g; Fiber: 3g; Total Fat: 7g

Chicken and Cheese Enchiladas

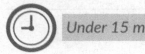 *Under 15 minutes*

INGREDIENTS:

» 2 small tortillas
» ½ cup cooked shredded chicken
» ¼ cup shredded cheese
» ¼ cup enchilada sauce

INSTRUCTIONS:

1. Preheat the oven to 400°F. Fill each tortilla with shredded chicken and cheese, then roll tightly and place seam-side down in a small baking dish.
2. Pour enchilada sauce over the top and sprinkle with remaining cheese.
3. Bake for 8-10 minutes until cheese is melted and bubbly. Serve warm. These quick enchiladas are filled with savory chicken and melted cheese, perfect for a satisfying and flavorful meal.

NUTRITIONAL VALUES (PER SERVING):

Calories: 280; Protein: 18g; Carbohydrates: 22g; Fiber: 2g; Total Fat: 14g

Pita Wraps with Tzatziki

 Under 15 minutes

INGREDIENTS:

» 1 whole wheat pita, halved
» ½ cup cucumber, diced
» 2 tablespoons tzatziki sauce
» ¼ cup cooked chicken or falafel

INSTRUCTIONS:

1. Spread tzatziki sauce inside each pita half, then add cucumber and chicken or falafel.
2. Press gently to ensure the fillings are evenly distributed.
3. Serve immediately for a refreshing, Mediterranean-inspired meal. These pita wraps are light, flavorful, and perfect for a quick lunch or dinner, packed with fresh veggies and creamy tzatziki.

NUTRITIONAL VALUES (PER SERVING):

Calories: 240; Protein: 12g; Carbohydrates: 30g; Fiber: 4g; Total Fat: 8g

Chickpea Curry

 Under 15 minutes

INGREDIENTS:

» 1 cup canned chickpeas, drained
» ¼ cup coconut milk
» 1 teaspoon curry powder

INSTRUCTIONS:

1. In a saucepan over medium heat, add chickpeas and coconut milk, stirring to combine.
2. Sprinkle in the curry powder and cook for 5-7 minutes, stirring occasionally, until the mixture is heated through and fragrant.
3. Serve over rice or with naan. This quick chickpea curry is creamy, aromatic, and packed with plant-based protein, making it a satisfying and flavorful meal.

NUTRITIONAL VALUES (PER SERVING):

Calories: 180; Protein: 6g; Carbohydrates: 24g; Fiber: 6g; Total Fat: 8g

Lemon Garlic Tilapia

 Under 15 minutes

INGREDIENTS:

- » 1 tilapia fillet
- » 1 tablespoon olive oil
- » 1 tablespoon lemon juice
- » 1 garlic clove, minced

INSTRUCTIONS:

1. In a skillet over medium heat, warm the olive oil and add minced garlic, cooking until fragrant.
2. Place the tilapia fillet in the skillet and drizzle with lemon juice. Cook for 3-4 minutes per side until the fish is flaky and cooked through.
3. Serve immediately with extra lemon wedges if desired. This light and zesty tilapia dish is quick to prepare and perfect for a refreshing, low-calorie meal.

NUTRITIONAL VALUES (PER SERVING):

Calories: 160; Protein: 20g; Carbohydrates: 1g; Fiber: 0g; Total Fat: 8g

Spaghetti Aglio e Olio

 Under 15 minutes

INGREDIENTS:

- » 1 cup cooked spaghetti
- » 2 tablespoons olive oil
- » 2 garlic cloves, thinly sliced
- » Red pepper flakes, to taste

INSTRUCTIONS:

1. In a skillet over medium heat, warm the olive oil and add garlic slices, cooking until golden and fragrant.
2. Add the cooked spaghetti and red pepper flakes, tossing to coat the pasta in the garlic-infused oil.
3. Serve immediately, garnished with parsley or Parmesan if desired. This simple Italian pasta dish is quick, flavorful, and made with minimal ingredients, offering a satisfying meal with a touch of heat.

NUTRITIONAL VALUES (PER SERVING):

Calories: 250; Protein: 6g; Carbohydrates: 42g; Fiber: 2g; Total Fat: 10g

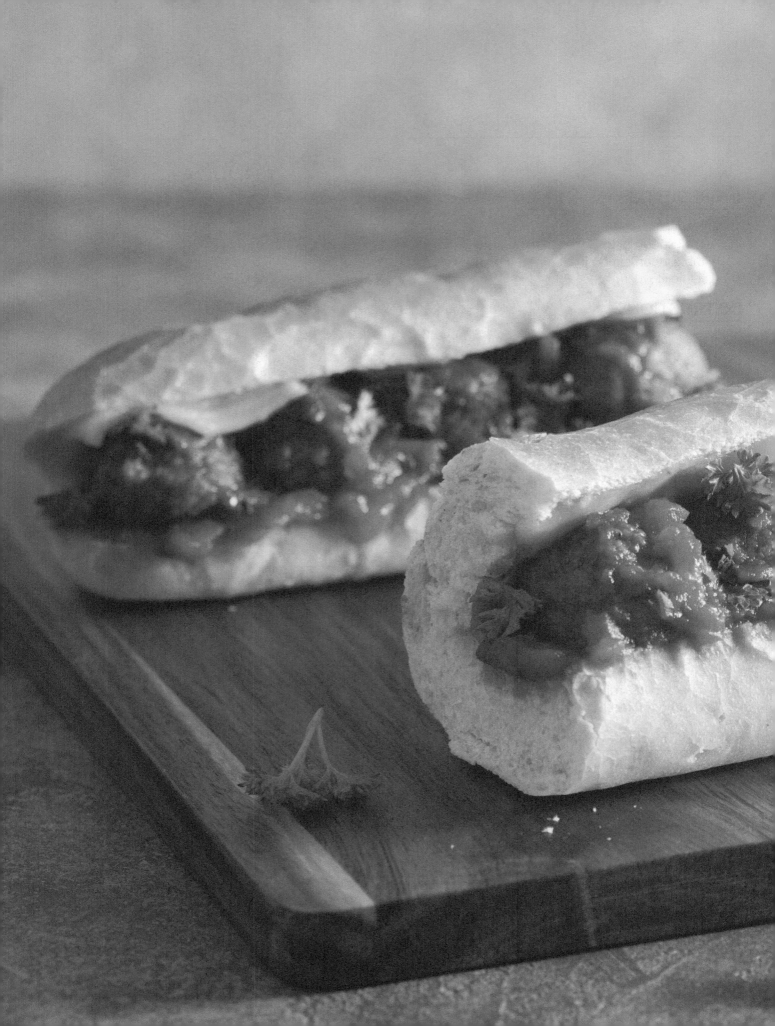

Chapter 3

20-MINUTE

Recipes

Fast meals for when you have just a bit more time.

Grilled Chicken with Pesto

 Under 20 minutes

INGREDIENTS:

» 1 boneless chicken breast
» 2 tablespoons pesto sauce
» 1 tablespoon olive oil

INSTRUCTIONS:

1. Heat olive oil in a skillet over medium heat. Add the chicken breast, cooking for 5-6 minutes per side until golden and cooked through.
2. Remove from heat and spoon pesto sauce over the chicken. Let it rest for a minute, allowing the pesto to warm and coat the chicken.
3. Slice and serve. This dish combines juicy grilled chicken with rich pesto, offering a quick yet elegant flavor-packed meal.

NUTRITIONAL VALUES (PER SERVING):

Calories: 250; Protein: 25g; Carbohydrates: 1g; Fiber: 0g; Total Fat: 15g

Shrimp Tacos with Avocado

 Under 20 minutes

INGREDIENTS:

» ½ cup shrimp, peeled and deveined
» 2 small corn tortillas
» ½ avocado, sliced
» 1 tablespoon lime juice

INSTRUCTIONS:

1. In a skillet over medium heat, cook the shrimp for 3-4 minutes until pink and cooked through.
2. Place shrimp and avocado slices onto the tortillas and drizzle with lime juice.
3. Serve with a sprinkle of cilantro or salsa if desired. These shrimp tacos are fresh, flavorful, and perfect for a light yet satisfying meal with a touch of zest.

NUTRITIONAL VALUES (PER SERVING):

Calories: 220; Protein: 14g; Carbohydrates: 18g; Fiber: 4g; Total Fat: 10g

Spaghetti with Meat Sauce

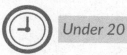 *Under 20 minutes*

INGREDIENTS:

» 1 cup cooked spaghetti
» ½ cup ground beef
» ¼ cup marinara sauce

INSTRUCTIONS:

1. In a skillet over medium heat, brown the ground beef, breaking it up as it cooks. Drain any excess fat.
2. Add marinara sauce to the skillet, stirring to combine with the beef. Let simmer for 5 minutes.
3. Toss with cooked spaghetti and serve warm. This classic spaghetti with meat sauce is quick, hearty, and packed with savory flavors, perfect for a filling meal.

NUTRITIONAL VALUES (PER SERVING):

Calories: 350; Protein: 18g; Carbohydrates: 40g; Fiber: 3g; Total Fat: 12g

Chicken Parmesan

 Under 20 minutes

INGREDIENTS:

» 1 boneless chicken breast
» ¼ cup marinara sauce
» 2 tablespoons shredded mozzarella

INSTRUCTIONS:

1. Cook the chicken breast in a skillet over medium heat for 5-6 minutes per side until golden and cooked through.
2. Spoon marinara sauce over the chicken, sprinkle with mozzarella, and cover for 2-3 minutes until the cheese melts.
3. Serve warm. This easy chicken Parmesan is cheesy, savory, and ideal for a quick Italian-inspired meal with minimal ingredients.

NUTRITIONAL VALUES (PER SERVING):

Calories: 300; Protein: 30g; Carbohydrates: 6g; Fiber: 1g; Total Fat: 15g

Mushroom Risotto

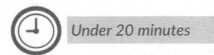 *Under 20 minutes*

INGREDIENTS:

» ½ cup Arborio rice
» 1 cup vegetable broth
» ¼ cup mushrooms, sliced

INSTRUCTIONS:

1. In a saucepan, heat vegetable broth to a simmer. In a separate skillet, cook mushrooms until tender.
2. Add Arborio rice to the skillet with mushrooms, stirring for 1-2 minutes. Gradually add broth, stirring until absorbed. Repeat until rice is creamy and tender, about 15 minutes.
3. Serve warm. This mushroom risotto is creamy, flavorful, and perfect for a comforting meal in a short time.

NUTRITIONAL VALUES (PER SERVING):

Calories: 240; Protein: 6g; Carbohydrates: 45g; Fiber: 2g; Total Fat: 5g

Turkey Burgers

 Under 20 minutes

INGREDIENTS:

» 1 turkey patty
» 1 whole-grain bun
» Lettuce and tomato slices

INSTRUCTIONS:

1. In a skillet, cook the turkey patty over medium heat for 5-6 minutes per side until cooked through.
2. Place on the bun and top with lettuce and tomato.
3. Serve warm with your favorite condiments. These lean turkey burgers are a quick, protein-packed meal, perfect for a healthier take on a classic burger.

NUTRITIONAL VALUES (PER SERVING):

Calories: 280; Protein: 25g; Carbohydrates: 30g; Fiber: 3g; Total Fat: 8g

Shrimp Fried Rice

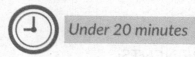 *Under 20 minutes*

INGREDIENTS:

- » ½ cup cooked rice
- » ¼ cup shrimp, peeled and deveined
- » 1 tablespoon soy sauce

INSTRUCTIONS:

1. In a skillet over medium heat, cook the shrimp until pink, about 3 minutes.
2. Add cooked rice and soy sauce, stirring to combine and heat through for 3-4 minutes.
3. Serve warm, garnished with green onions if desired. This quick shrimp fried rice is savory and satisfying, packed with protein and flavor.

NUTRITIONAL VALUES (PER SERVING):

Calories: 230; Protein: 12g; Carbohydrates: 30g; Fiber: 2g; Total Fat: 6g

Chicken Piccata

 Under 20 minutes

INGREDIENTS:

- » 1 boneless chicken breast
- » 1 tablespoon lemon juice
- » 1 tablespoon capers

INSTRUCTIONS:

1. Cook the chicken breast in a skillet over medium heat for 5-6 minutes per side until golden and cooked through.
2. Add lemon juice and capers to the skillet, cooking for an additional 2 minutes to infuse flavors.
3. Serve warm with a garnish of parsley if desired. This chicken piccata is tangy and delicious, perfect for a quick, elegant meal.

NUTRITIONAL VALUES (PER SERVING):

Calories: 220; Protein: 24g; Carbohydrates: 2g; Fiber: 0g; Total Fat: 12g

Thai Peanut Noodles

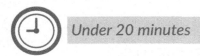 *Under 20 minutes*

INGREDIENTS:

» 1 cup cooked noodles
» 1 tablespoon peanut butter
» 1 tablespoon soy sauce

INSTRUCTIONS:

1. In a small bowl, mix peanut butter and soy sauce until smooth.
2. Toss with warm noodles until well coated.
3. Serve garnished with chopped green onions or peanuts if desired. These Thai peanut noodles are creamy, nutty, and flavorful, making a quick and satisfying meal with minimal ingredients.

NUTRITIONAL VALUES (PER SERVING):

Calories: 260; Protein: 8g; Carbohydrates: 40g; Fiber: 3g; Total Fat: 10g

Chicken Pot Pie

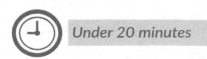 *Under 20 minutes*

INGREDIENTS:

» ½ cup cooked chicken, shredded
» ¼ cup mixed vegetables (peas, carrots)
» ¼ cup chicken broth
» 1 refrigerated biscuit

INSTRUCTIONS:

1. In a skillet, combine chicken, vegetables, and chicken broth, cooking until heated through.
2. Place the mixture in a small baking dish and top with the biscuit.
3. Bake at 375°F for 10-12 minutes until the biscuit is golden. This quick chicken pot pie is hearty and comforting, perfect for a speedy homemade meal.

NUTRITIONAL VALUES (PER SERVING):

Calories: 280; Protein: 15g; Carbohydrates: 30g; Fiber: 3g; Total Fat: 10g

Vegetarian Paella

 Under 20 minutes

INGREDIENTS:

- » ½ cup Arborio or short-grain rice
- » ¼ cup bell peppers, diced
- » ¼ cup peas
- » 1 cup vegetable broth

INSTRUCTIONS:

1. In a large skillet, combine vegetable broth, rice, and bell peppers, bringing to a simmer.
2. Cook for about 15 minutes, stirring occasionally, until the rice absorbs the broth and becomes tender.
3. Stir in peas and cook for an additional 3 minutes. Serve warm, garnished with parsley. This vegetarian paella is rich in flavors, bringing Spanish-inspired tastes to a quick, nutritious meal.

NUTRITIONAL VALUES (PER SERVING):

Calories: 200; Protein: 5g; Carbohydrates: 40g; Fiber: 3g; Total Fat: 3g

Baked Salmon with Garlic Butter

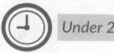 *Under 20 minutes*

INGREDIENTS:

- » 1 salmon fillet (4 oz)
- » 1 tablespoon butter, melted
- » 1 garlic clove, minced

INSTRUCTIONS:

1. Preheat oven to 400°F. Place the salmon on a baking sheet and brush with melted butter and garlic.
2. Bake for 10-12 minutes until the salmon flakes easily with a fork.
3. Serve warm with lemon wedges if desired. This baked salmon is tender and flavorful, perfect for a quick and healthy dinner.

NUTRITIONAL VALUES (PER SERVING):

Calories: 250; Protein: 22g; Carbohydrates: 1g; Fiber: 0g; Total Fat: 18g

Mexican Rice Bowls

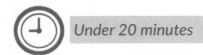 *Under 20 minutes*

INGREDIENTS:

» ½ cup cooked rice
» ¼ cup black beans
» ¼ cup corn
» 2 tablespoons salsa

INSTRUCTIONS:

1. In a bowl, layer the cooked rice, black beans, and corn.
2. Top with salsa, and garnish with cilantro if desired.
3. Serve warm for a quick, flavorful Mexican-inspired bowl packed with protein and fiber. This dish is versatile and customizable, ideal for a balanced and filling meal.

NUTRITIONAL VALUES (PER SERVING):

Calories: 220; Protein: 8g; Carbohydrates: 40g; Fiber: 6g; Total Fat: 4g

Tuna Casserole

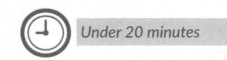 *Under 20 minutes*

INGREDIENTS:

» ½ cup cooked pasta
» 1 can tuna, drained (5 oz)
» ¼ cup cream of mushroom soup

INSTRUCTIONS:

1. In a baking dish, combine the pasta, tuna, and cream of mushroom soup, mixing until evenly coated.
2. Bake at 375°F for 10-12 minutes until warmed through.
3. Serve hot, optionally topped with breadcrumbs. This tuna casserole is creamy, comforting, and perfect for a quick family meal.

NUTRITIONAL VALUES (PER SERVING):

Calories: 300; Protein: 20g; Carbohydrates: 30g; Fiber: 2g; Total Fat: 12g

Spinach and Cheese Lasagna

 Under 20 minutes

INGREDIENTS:

» 2 lasagna noodles, cooked
» ¼ cup ricotta cheese
» ½ cup spinach, chopped

INSTRUCTIONS:

1. Preheat oven to 375°F. Layer one noodle with ricotta cheese and spinach, then top with the second noodle.
2. Bake for 10-12 minutes until heated through and cheese is melted.
3. Serve warm. This simplified lasagna is cheesy, comforting, and packed with spinach, making it a quick, nutritious option.

NUTRITIONAL VALUES (PER SERVING):

Calories: 220; Protein: 12g; Carbohydrates: 28g; Fiber: 4g; Total Fat: 8g

Meatball Subs

 Under 20 minutes

INGREDIENTS:

» 2 small sandwich rolls
» 4 pre-cooked meatballs
» ¼ cup marinara sauce

INSTRUCTIONS:

1. In a saucepan, heat the marinara sauce and meatballs until warm, about 5 minutes.
2. Place two meatballs in each roll and spoon marinara sauce over the top.
3. Serve immediately, optionally topped with grated Parmesan. These meatball subs are savory and satisfying, perfect for a quick, hearty meal.

NUTRITIONAL VALUES (PER SERVING):

Calories: 300; Protein: 18g; Carbohydrates: 32g; Fiber: 2g; Total Fat: 12g

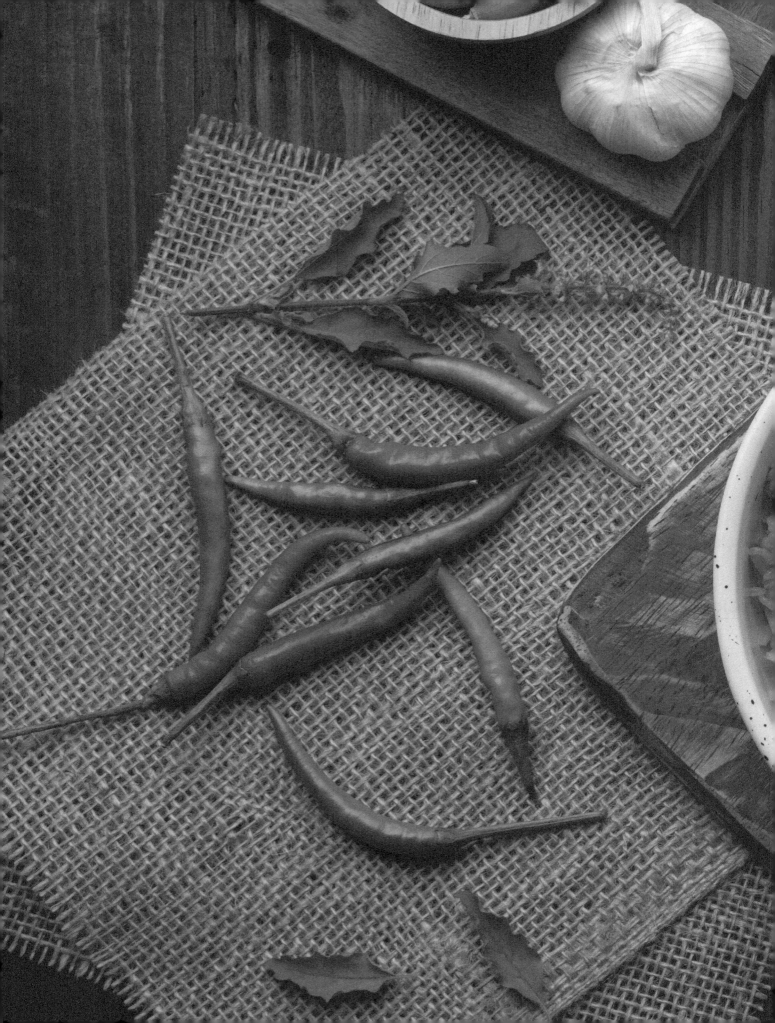

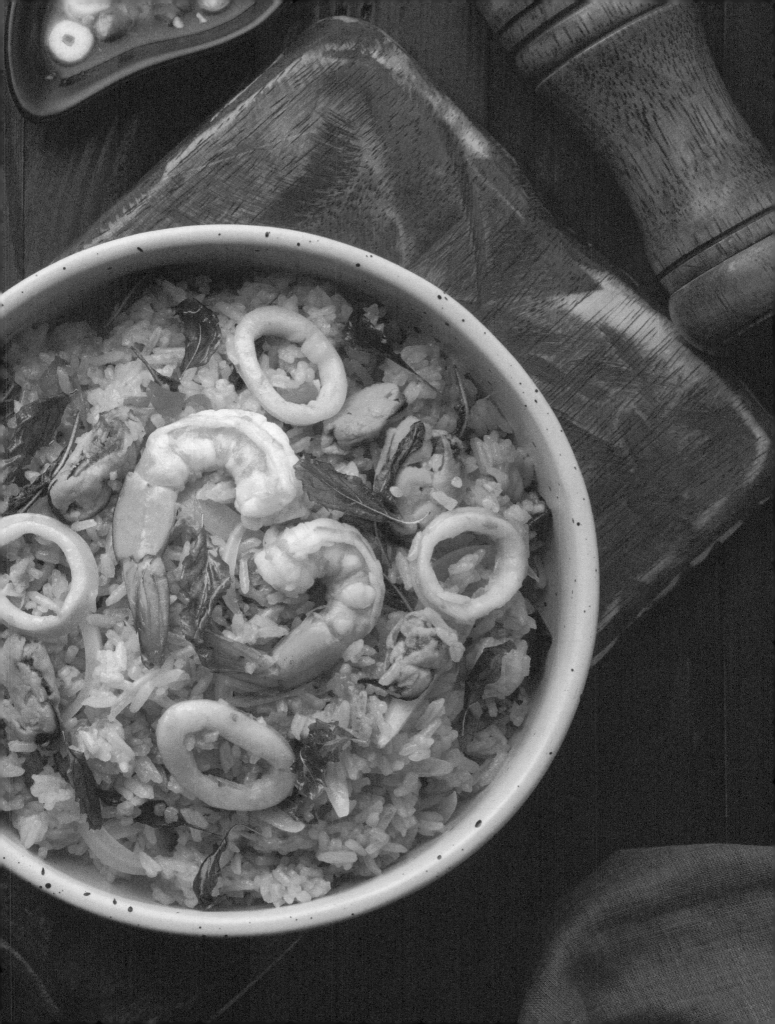

Grilled Chicken with Mango Salsa

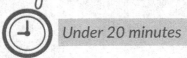 *Under 20 minutes*

INGREDIENTS:

» 1 chicken breast, grilled
» ¼ cup diced mango
» 1 tablespoon cilantro, chopped

INSTRUCTIONS:

1. Grill the chicken breast over medium heat for 6-8 minutes per side until cooked through.
2. In a bowl, combine diced mango and cilantro, and spoon over the grilled chicken.
3. Serve immediately. The sweet mango salsa complements the grilled chicken perfectly, creating a refreshing, tropical-inspired dish.

NUTRITIONAL VALUES (PER SERVING):

Calories: 240; Protein: 25g; Carbohydrates: 12g; Fiber: 2g; Total Fat: 8g

Spaghetti Bolognese

 Under 20 minutes

INGREDIENTS:

» 1 cup cooked spaghetti
» ¼ cup ground beef, cooked
» ¼ cup marinara sauce

INSTRUCTIONS:

1. In a saucepan, combine cooked ground beef and marinara sauce, heating until warm.
2. Toss with cooked spaghetti until evenly coated.
3. Serve warm with Parmesan cheese if desired. This classic spaghetti Bolognese is quick, rich in flavor, and perfect for a hearty meal.

NUTRITIONAL VALUES (PER SERVING):

Calories: 340; Protein: 18g; Carbohydrates: 42g; Fiber: 3g; Total Fat: 12g

Chicken Burrito Bowl

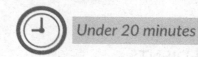 *Under 20 minutes*

INGREDIENTS:

» ½ cup cooked rice
» ¼ cup cooked chicken breast, diced
» ¼ cup black beans
» 2 tablespoons salsa

INSTRUCTIONS:

1. In a bowl, layer the rice, chicken, black beans, and salsa.
2. Garnish with cilantro or shredded cheese if desired.
3. Serve warm. This chicken burrito bowl is hearty and customizable, filled with protein and fresh flavors for a satisfying meal.

NUTRITIONAL VALUES (PER SERVING):

Calories: 260; Protein: 20g; Carbohydrates: 36g; Fiber: 6g; Total Fat: 6g

Gnocchi with Sage Butter

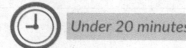 *Under 20 minutes*

INGREDIENTS:

» 1 cup cooked gnocchi
» 1 tablespoon butter
» 2 sage leaves, chopped

INSTRUCTIONS:

1. In a skillet over medium heat, melt butter and add sage leaves, cooking until butter is lightly browned and fragrant.
2. Toss in the gnocchi, stirring until evenly coated in sage butter.
3. Serve immediately with grated Parmesan if desired. This simple gnocchi dish is buttery, aromatic, and ready in minutes, ideal for a quick, comforting meal.

NUTRITIONAL VALUES (PER SERVING):

Calories: 280; Protein: 6g; Carbohydrates: 40g; Fiber: 2g; Total Fat: 10g

Chicken and Mushroom Stroganoff

 Under 20 minutes

INGREDIENTS:

» 1 boneless chicken breast, sliced
» ¼ cup mushrooms, sliced
» ¼ cup sour cream
» 1 tablespoon olive oil

INSTRUCTIONS:

1. In a skillet over medium heat, warm the olive oil. Add chicken and mushrooms, cooking until the chicken is fully cooked and the mushrooms are tender, about 6-8 minutes.
2. Reduce heat to low, stir in the sour cream, and let it simmer for 2-3 minutes until creamy.
3. Serve over pasta or rice for a comforting, creamy meal. This quick stroganoff offers tender chicken and rich flavors in a short time.

NUTRITIONAL VALUES (PER SERVING):

Calories: 250; Protein: 20g; Carbohydrates: 6g; Fiber: 1g; Total Fat: 16g

Prawn Stir-Fry

 Under 20 minutes

INGREDIENTS:

» ½ cup prawns, peeled and deveined
» ½ cup mixed vegetables (bell peppers, broccoli)
» 1 tablespoon soy sauce
» 1 tablespoon olive oil

INSTRUCTIONS:

1. In a skillet over medium-high heat, add olive oil and prawns, cooking for 2-3 minutes until pink.
2. Add mixed vegetables and soy sauce, stir-frying until vegetables are tender-crisp, about 5 minutes.
3. Serve hot, garnished with green onions if desired. This prawn stir-fry is packed with flavors and provides a quick, nutritious meal filled with protein and veggies.

NUTRITIONAL VALUES (PER SERVING):

Calories: 180; Protein: 16g; Carbohydrates: 8g; Fiber: 2g; Total Fat: 8g

Italian Beef Sandwiches

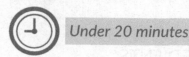 *Under 20 minutes*

INGREDIENTS:

» ½ cup shredded cooked beef
» ¼ cup marinara sauce
» 1 small sandwich roll

INSTRUCTIONS:

1. In a skillet, heat the shredded beef and marinara sauce until warmed through, about 5 minutes.
2. Spoon the beef mixture onto the sandwich roll.
3. Serve warm, optionally topped with provolone cheese for an extra savory kick. This Italian beef sandwich is hearty and flavorful, offering a delicious meal option with minimal prep time.

NUTRITIONAL VALUES (PER SERVING):

Calories: 280; Protein: 18g; Carbohydrates: 25g; Fiber: 2g; Total Fat: 12g

Cauliflower Mac and Cheese

 Under 20 minutes

INGREDIENTS:

» 1 cup cauliflower florets
» ¼ cup shredded cheddar cheese
» ¼ cup milk

INSTRUCTIONS:

1. Steam cauliflower florets until tender, about 5-7 minutes.
2. In a saucepan over low heat, combine milk and cheddar cheese, stirring until melted.
3. Toss in the steamed cauliflower until coated. Serve hot for a low-carb twist on traditional mac and cheese that's creamy and satisfying.

NUTRITIONAL VALUES (PER SERVING):

Calories: 150; Protein: 8g; Carbohydrates: 10g; Fiber: 3g; Total Fat: 10g

Bbq Pulled Pork Sandwiches

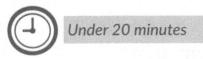 *Under 20 minutes*

INGREDIENTS:

» ½ cup cooked shredded pork
» 2 tablespoons BBQ sauce
» 1 small sandwich roll

INSTRUCTIONS:

1. In a skillet, heat shredded pork and BBQ sauce until warm and evenly coated, about 5 minutes.
2. Spoon the pork onto the sandwich roll and serve immediately.
3. Optionally, add coleslaw for a tangy crunch. This pulled pork sandwich is packed with smoky, savory flavors and is perfect for a quick and satisfying meal.

NUTRITIONAL VALUES (PER SERVING):

Calories: 300; Protein: 15g; Carbohydrates: 25g; Fiber: 2g; Total Fat: 15g

Shrimp Alfredo Pasta

 Under 20 minutes

INGREDIENTS:

» ½ cup cooked pasta
» ¼ cup shrimp, peeled and deveined
» ¼ cup Alfredo sauce

INSTRUCTIONS:

1. In a skillet, cook the shrimp over medium heat for 3-4 minutes until pink.
2. Add cooked pasta and Alfredo sauce, stirring to coat evenly.
3. Serve hot, garnished with parsley if desired. This creamy shrimp Alfredo is rich and satisfying, making it an ideal choice for a quick and comforting dinner.

NUTRITIONAL VALUES (PER SERVING):

Calories: 280; Protein: 14g; Carbohydrates: 30g; Fiber: 2g; Total Fat: 12g

Vegan Tofu Scramble

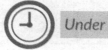 *Under 20 minutes*

INGREDIENTS:

- » ½ cup firm tofu, crumbled
- » ¼ cup bell peppers, diced
- » 1 tablespoon nutritional yeast

INSTRUCTIONS:

1. In a skillet, cook crumbled tofu and bell peppers over medium heat for 5-7 minutes until peppers are tender.
2. Stir in nutritional yeast for a cheesy flavor and season with salt and pepper.
3. Serve warm. This vegan tofu scramble is high in protein and offers a delicious, plant-based alternative to scrambled eggs.

NUTRITIONAL VALUES (PER SERVING):

Calories: 120; Protein: 10g; Carbohydrates: 5g; Fiber: 2g; Total Fat: 7g

Pork Chops with Applesauce

Under 20 minutes

INGREDIENTS:

- » 1 pork chop
- » ¼ cup unsweetened applesauce
- » Salt and pepper to taste

INSTRUCTIONS:

1. In a skillet over medium heat, cook the pork chop for 4-5 minutes per side until browned and cooked through.
2. Serve with a side of applesauce, seasoned with salt and pepper if desired.
3. This dish offers a savory and sweet combination, perfect for a quick, balanced meal.

NUTRITIONAL VALUES (PER SERVING):

Calories: 240; Protein: 22g; Carbohydrates: 8g; Fiber: 1g; Total Fat: 12g

Greek Lemon Chicken Soup

 Under 20 minutes

INGREDIENTS:

» 1 cup chicken broth
» ¼ cup cooked chicken, shredded
» 1 tablespoon lemon juice

INSTRUCTIONS:

1. In a saucepan, combine chicken broth, shredded chicken, and lemon juice.
2. Simmer for 5-7 minutes until heated through.
3. Serve hot, garnished with fresh dill or parsley. This Greek-inspired soup is light, tangy, and perfect for a quick, nourishing meal.

NUTRITIONAL VALUES (PER SERVING):

Calories: 80; Protein: 10g; Carbohydrates: 2g; Fiber: 0g; Total Fat: 3g

Chicken Fajitas

 Under 20 minutes

INGREDIENTS:

» ½ cup chicken breast, sliced
» ½ cup bell peppers, sliced
» 1 tablespoon fajita seasoning

INSTRUCTIONS:

1. In a skillet over medium-high heat, cook chicken and bell peppers with fajita seasoning for about 5-7 minutes until the chicken is cooked through and peppers are tender.
2. Serve in warm tortillas, garnished with salsa or sour cream if desired.
3. These chicken fajitas are flavorful and colorful, making for a quick and satisfying Tex-Mex meal.

NUTRITIONAL VALUES (PER SERVING):

Calories: 250; Protein: 20g; Carbohydrates: 12g; Fiber: 2g; Total Fat: 12g

Baked Potato with Bacon

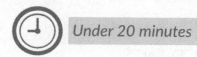 *Under 20 minutes*

INGREDIENTS:

» 1 large potato
» 2 slices bacon, cooked and crumbled
» 1 tablespoon sour cream

INSTRUCTIONS:

1. Microwave the potato on high for 5-7 minutes until soft, then carefully slice open and fluff with a fork.
2. Sprinkle the crumbled bacon over the potato and add a dollop of sour cream.
3. Serve hot, optionally garnished with chives. This baked potato with bacon is hearty, warm, and packed with flavor, making it a quick and satisfying side or meal.

NUTRITIONAL VALUES (PER SERVING):

Calories: 220; Protein: 6g; Carbohydrates: 35g; Fiber: 4g; Total Fat: 8g

Eggplant Parmesan

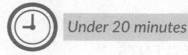 *Under 20 minutes*

INGREDIENTS:

» 1 small eggplant, sliced
» ¼ cup marinara sauce
» 2 tablespoons shredded mozzarella cheese

INSTRUCTIONS:

1. Preheat the oven to 400°F. Place eggplant slices on a baking sheet, spoon marinara sauce over each slice, and sprinkle with mozzarella.
2. Bake for 10-12 minutes until the cheese is melted and bubbly.
3. Serve warm. This quick Eggplant Parmesan is a lighter version of the classic, offering savory flavors and cheesy goodness in a short time.

NUTRITIONAL VALUES (PER SERVING):

Calories: 160; Protein: 5g; Carbohydrates: 10g; Fiber: 4g; Total Fat: 10g

Sesame Ginger Chicken

 Under 20 minutes

INGREDIENTS:

» 1 chicken breast, diced
» 1 tablespoon sesame oil
» 1 teaspoon fresh ginger, grated

INSTRUCTIONS:

1. In a skillet over medium heat, add sesame oil and cook chicken with ginger, stirring until golden and cooked through, about 8-10 minutes.
2. Serve hot, garnished with sesame seeds if desired. This sesame ginger chicken is aromatic and full of flavor, providing a quick and delicious meal with an Asian-inspired twist.

NUTRITIONAL VALUES (PER SERVING):

Calories: 220; Protein: 25g; Carbohydrates: 2g; Fiber: 0g; Total Fat: 12g

Beef Ragu

 Under 20 minutes

INGREDIENTS:

» ½ cup ground beef
» ¼ cup diced tomatoes
» 1 teaspoon Italian seasoning

INSTRUCTIONS:

1. In a skillet, cook ground beef over medium heat until browned. Drain excess fat.
2. Add diced tomatoes and Italian seasoning, simmering for 5-7 minutes until thickened.
3. Serve over pasta or polenta. This quick beef ragu is hearty and rich, perfect for a fast, comforting meal with minimal ingredients.

NUTRITIONAL VALUES (PER SERVING):

Calories: 250; Protein: 18g; Carbohydrates: 4g; Fiber: 1g; Total Fat: 18g

Butternut Squash Soup

 Under 20 minutes

INGREDIENTS:

» 1 cup butternut squash, cubed
» 1 cup vegetable broth
» 1 tablespoon cream

INSTRUCTIONS:

1. In a pot, combine butternut squash and vegetable broth, bringing to a boil. Simmer for 10 minutes until squash is tender.
2. Use an immersion blender to purée until smooth, then stir in cream.
3. Serve warm. This creamy butternut squash soup is comforting, sweet, and perfect for a quick, nutritious meal.

NUTRITIONAL VALUES (PER SERVING):

Calories: 120; Protein: 2g; Carbohydrates: 20g; Fiber: 3g; Total Fat: 4g

Chicken Marsala

 Under 20 minutes

INGREDIENTS:

» 1 boneless chicken breast
» ¼ cup mushrooms, sliced
» ¼ cup Marsala wine

INSTRUCTIONS:

1. In a skillet, cook the chicken breast over medium heat until browned, about 5 minutes per side. Remove and set aside.
2. Add mushrooms to the skillet and cook until softened, then add Marsala wine, simmering for 3-5 minutes.
3. Return chicken to the skillet, coating with sauce, and serve. This Chicken Marsala is elegant, flavorful, and perfect for a quick, satisfying meal.

NUTRITIONAL VALUES (PER SERVING):

Calories: 240; Protein: 25g; Carbohydrates: 5g; Fiber: 1g; Total Fat: 10g

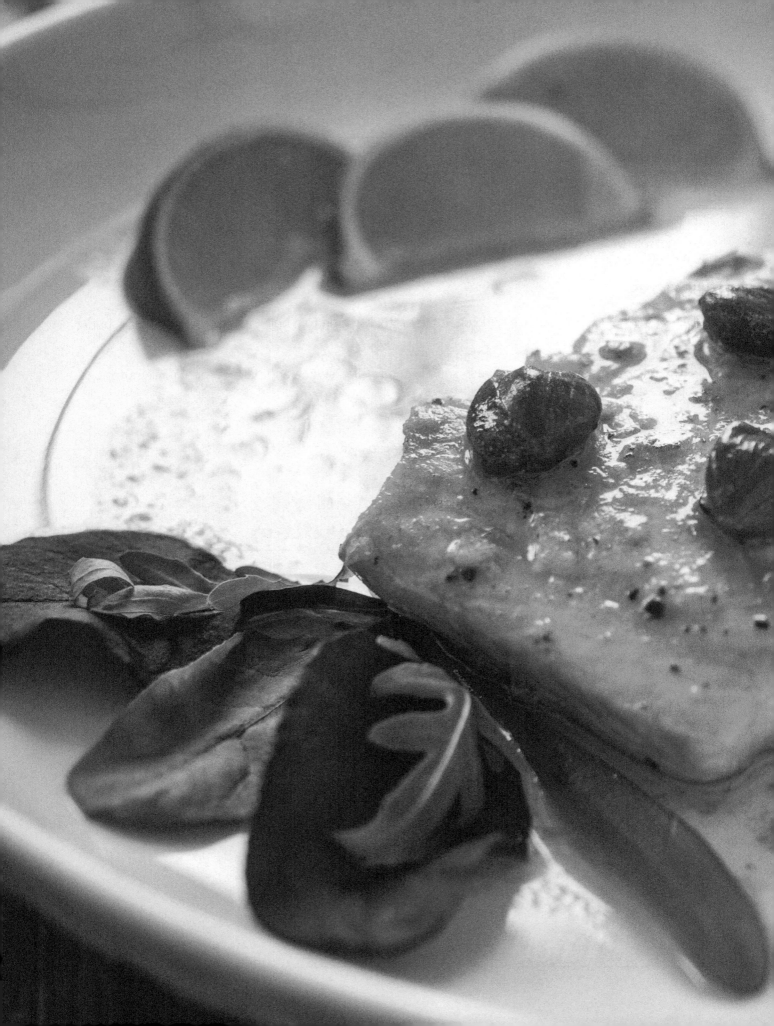

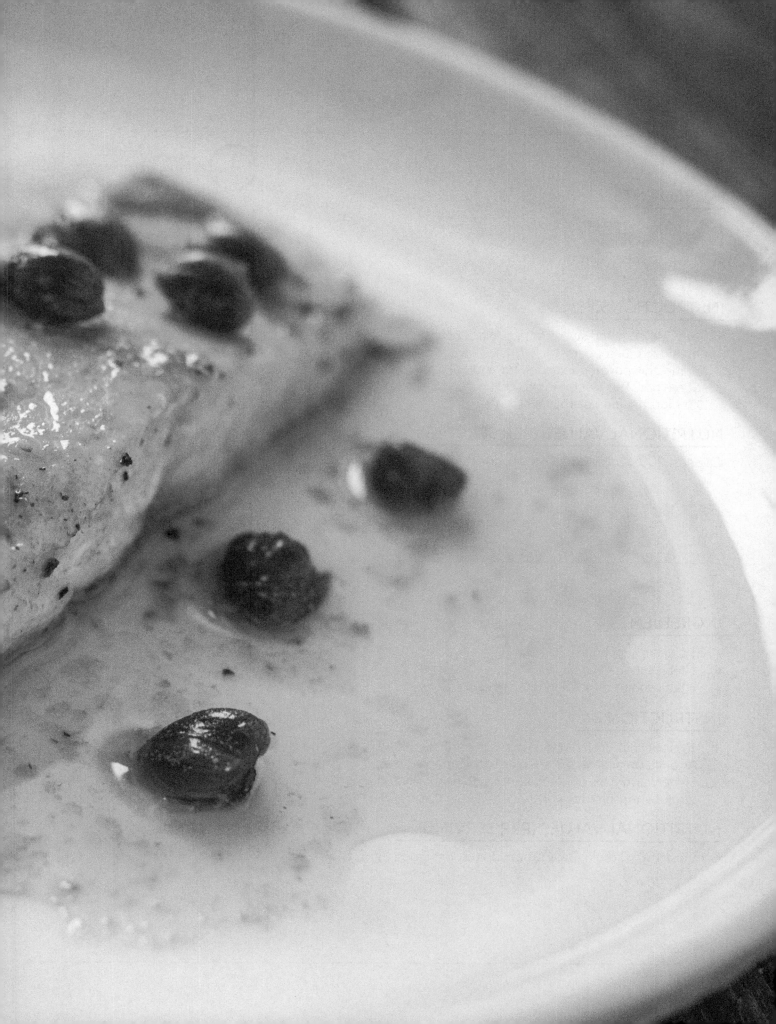

Sweet Potato Chili

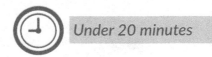 *Under 20 minutes*

INGREDIENTS:

» 1 cup sweet potato, cubed
» ½ cup black beans
» 1 cup vegetable broth
» 1 teaspoon chili powder

INSTRUCTIONS:

1. In a pot, combine sweet potato, black beans, and vegetable broth, simmering over medium heat for 15 minutes until tender.
2. Stir in chili powder and cook for another 2 minutes.
3. Serve hot. This sweet potato chili is hearty, spicy, and packed with plant-based goodness, perfect for a comforting and healthy meal.

NUTRITIONAL VALUES (PER SERVING):

Calories: 200; Protein: 6g; Carbohydrates: 35g; Fiber: 8g; Total Fat: 2g

Grilled Zucchini with Feta

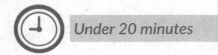 *Under 20 minutes*

INGREDIENTS:

» 1 zucchini, sliced
» 1 tablespoon olive oil
» 2 tablespoons crumbled feta cheese

INSTRUCTIONS:

1. Toss zucchini slices with olive oil and grill over medium heat for 3-4 minutes per side until tender.
2. Arrange on a plate and sprinkle with crumbled feta.
3. Serve warm. This quick, flavorful side dish pairs tender grilled zucchini with salty feta for a refreshing Mediterranean-inspired flavor.

NUTRITIONAL VALUES (PER SERVING):

Calories: 100; Protein: 3g; Carbohydrates: 6g; Fiber: 2g; Total Fat: 8g

Moroccan Lamb Stew

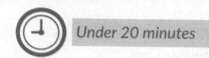
Under 20 minutes

INGREDIENTS:

- » ½ cup diced lamb
- » ¼ cup chickpeas
- » ½ cup vegetable broth
- » 1 teaspoon cumin

INSTRUCTIONS:

1. In a pot, combine lamb, chickpeas, and vegetable broth, bringing to a simmer.
2. Add cumin and cook for 15 minutes until lamb is tender and flavors are infused.
3. Serve warm. This Moroccan lamb stew is rich, spiced, and quick to make, offering a taste of North Africa in a comforting dish.

NUTRITIONAL VALUES (PER SERVING):

Calories: 250; Protein: 18g; Carbohydrates: 12g; Fiber: 3g; Total Fat: 15g

Creamy Tomato Pasta

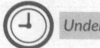
Under 20 minutes

INGREDIENTS:

- » 1 cup cooked pasta
- » ¼ cup tomato sauce
- » 2 tablespoons cream

INSTRUCTIONS:

1. In a saucepan, combine tomato sauce and cream, stirring until smooth. Heat over medium for 3-5 minutes.
2. Toss in cooked pasta, stirring until evenly coated.
3. Serve warm, garnished with basil if desired. This creamy tomato pasta is rich, comforting, and perfect for a quick Italian-inspired meal with minimal ingredients.

NUTRITIONAL VALUES (PER SERVING):

Calories: 280; Protein: 7g; Carbohydrates: 40g; Fiber: 3g; Total Fat: 10g

Lemon Garlic Chicken Thighs

 Under 20 minutes

INGREDIENTS:

» 2 chicken thighs
» 1 tablespoon olive oil
» 1 tablespoon lemon juice
» 1 garlic clove, minced

INSTRUCTIONS:

1. In a skillet, heat olive oil over medium heat. Add chicken thighs, cooking for 5-6 minutes per side until browned and cooked through.
2. Drizzle with lemon juice and add minced garlic in the final 2 minutes of cooking, stirring to coat.
3. Serve warm. These lemon garlic chicken thighs are zesty and flavorful, perfect for a quick, satisfying meal with minimal ingredients.

NUTRITIONAL VALUES (PER SERVING):

Calories: 220; Protein: 18g; Carbohydrates: 1g; Fiber: 0g; Total Fat: 16g

Vegetarian Chili

 Under 20 minutes

INGREDIENTS:

» ½ cup black beans
» ½ cup kidney beans
» 1 cup diced tomatoes
» 1 teaspoon chili powder

INSTRUCTIONS:

1. In a pot, combine black beans, kidney beans, diced tomatoes, and chili powder.
2. Simmer over medium heat for 10-15 minutes, stirring occasionally.
3. Serve warm, optionally garnished with sour cream or shredded cheese. This vegetarian chili is hearty, spicy, and perfect for a quick, protein-packed meal that's both filling and nutritious.

NUTRITIONAL VALUES (PER SERVING):

Calories: 180; Protein: 8g; Carbohydrates: 30g; Fiber: 8g; Total Fat: 2g

Chicken Caesar Wrap

 Under 20 minutes

INGREDIENTS:

- » 1 large tortilla
- » ½ cup cooked chicken, sliced
- » 2 tablespoons Caesar dressing
- » ¼ cup romaine lettuce, chopped

INSTRUCTIONS:

1. Lay the tortilla flat and spread Caesar dressing over it.
2. Add chicken and romaine lettuce, then roll up the tortilla tightly.
3. Slice in half and serve. This chicken Caesar wrap is a fresh and easy option for a quick lunch or light dinner, providing protein and classic Caesar flavors in a portable format.

NUTRITIONAL VALUES (PER SERVING):

Calories: 300; Protein: 20g; Carbohydrates: 30g; Fiber: 3g; Total Fat: 10g

Sausage and Pepper Skillet

 Under 20 minutes

INGREDIENTS:

- » 1 sausage link, sliced
- » ½ cup bell peppers, sliced
- » 1 tablespoon olive oil

INSTRUCTIONS:

1. In a skillet over medium heat, add olive oil and cook sausage slices until browned.
2. Add bell peppers, stirring until tender, about 5 minutes.
3. Serve hot. This sausage and pepper skillet is savory, colorful, and packed with flavor, perfect for a quick and hearty meal with minimal prep time.

NUTRITIONAL VALUES (PER SERVING):

Calories: 250; Protein: 12g; Carbohydrates: 8g; Fiber: 2g; Total Fat: 18g

Pork Loin with Cranberry Sauce

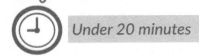 *Under 20 minutes*

INGREDIENTS:

» 1 pork loin chop
» ¼ cup cranberry sauce
» Salt and pepper to taste

INSTRUCTIONS:

1. In a skillet over medium heat, cook pork loin chop for 4-5 minutes per side until browned and cooked through.
2. Spoon cranberry sauce over the pork, warming for an additional minute.
3. Serve immediately. This pork loin with cranberry sauce is sweet and savory, offering a quick and elegant meal perfect for any time of year.

NUTRITIONAL VALUES (PER SERVING):

Calories: 240; Protein: 20g; Carbohydrates: 12g; Fiber: 1g; Total Fat: 10g

Chicken Alfredo Pizza

 Under 20 minutes

INGREDIENTS:

» 1 small pizza crust
» ¼ cup Alfredo sauce
» ½ cup cooked chicken, shredded
» ¼ cup mozzarella cheese

INSTRUCTIONS:

1. Preheat the oven to 400°F. Spread Alfredo sauce over the pizza crust, then top with shredded chicken and mozzarella cheese.
2. Bake for 10-12 minutes until cheese is melted and bubbly.
3. Serve warm. This chicken Alfredo pizza is creamy, cheesy, and perfect for a quick meal with comforting flavors.

NUTRITIONAL VALUES (PER SERVING):

Calories: 300; Protein: 20g; Carbohydrates: 25g; Fiber: 2g; Total Fat: 12g

Baked Tilapia with Lemon Butter

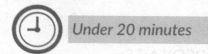 *Under 20 minutes*

INGREDIENTS:

- » 1 tilapia fillet
- » 1 tablespoon butter, melted
- » 1 teaspoon lemon juice

INSTRUCTIONS:

1. Preheat oven to 400°F. Place the tilapia on a baking sheet and drizzle with melted butter and lemon juice.
2. Bake for 10-12 minutes until the fish flakes easily with a fork.
3. Serve warm with additional lemon wedges if desired. This baked tilapia is light, flavorful, and ideal for a quick, healthy meal.

NUTRITIONAL VALUES (PER SERVING):

Calories: 160; Protein: 22g; Carbohydrates: 1g; Fiber: 0g; Total Fat: 8g

Mushroom Stroganoff

 Under 20 minutes

INGREDIENTS:

- » 1 cup mushrooms, sliced
- » ¼ cup sour cream
- » ½ cup vegetable broth
- » 1 tablespoon butter

INSTRUCTIONS:

1. In a skillet over medium heat, melt the butter and cook mushrooms until tender.
2. Add vegetable broth and simmer for 5 minutes, then stir in sour cream.
3. Serve warm over pasta or rice. This mushroom stroganoff is creamy and comforting, making it a quick, hearty option for a vegetarian meal.

NUTRITIONAL VALUES (PER SERVING):

Calories: 180; Protein: 4g; Carbohydrates: 10g; Fiber: 2g; Total Fat: 12g

Veggie Tacos

 Under 20 minutes

INGREDIENTS:

» 2 small corn tortillas
» ½ cup black beans
» ¼ cup bell peppers, diced
» 1 tablespoon salsa

INSTRUCTIONS:

1. Warm the tortillas in a skillet, then fill with black beans, bell peppers, and a spoonful of salsa.
2. Serve immediately, garnished with cilantro if desired.
3. These veggie tacos are light, fresh, and packed with flavor, making for a quick and nutritious meal with minimal ingredients.

NUTRITIONAL VALUES (PER SERVING):

Calories: 180; Protein: 6g; Carbohydrates: 26g; Fiber: 5g; Total Fat: 4g

Beef and Barley Soup

Under 20 minutes

INGREDIENTS:

» ½ cup cooked ground beef
» ¼ cup barley, cooked
» 1 cup beef broth

INSTRUCTIONS:

1. In a pot, combine cooked ground beef, barley, and beef broth, simmering for 10 minutes over medium heat until warmed through.
2. Season with salt and pepper and serve hot.
3. This beef and barley soup is hearty, savory, and perfect for a quick, comforting meal that's both filling and flavorful.

NUTRITIONAL VALUES (PER SERVING):

Calories: 200; Protein: 12g; Carbohydrates: 20g; Fiber: 3g; Total Fat: 8g

Grilled Chicken Salad

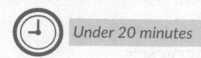 *Under 20 minutes*

INGREDIENTS:

- » 1 grilled chicken breast, sliced
- » 2 cups mixed greens
- » ¼ cup cherry tomatoes, halved
- » 2 tablespoons vinaigrette dressing

INSTRUCTIONS:

1. In a large bowl, combine mixed greens and cherry tomatoes.
2. Add sliced grilled chicken on top and drizzle with vinaigrette dressing.
3. Serve immediately. This grilled chicken salad is light, refreshing, and packed with protein, making it an ideal option for a quick and healthy meal.

NUTRITIONAL VALUES (PER SERVING):

Calories: 220; Protein: 20g; Carbohydrates: 6g; Fiber: 3g; Total Fat: 12g

Bbq Pulled Chicken

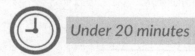 *Under 20 minutes*

INGREDIENTS:

- » ½ cup cooked shredded chicken
- » 2 tablespoons BBQ sauce
- » 1 small sandwich roll

INSTRUCTIONS:

1. In a skillet over medium heat, combine shredded chicken and BBQ sauce, stirring until heated through.
2. Spoon the mixture onto a sandwich roll and serve hot.
3. This BBQ pulled chicken is savory and smoky, perfect for a quick, filling sandwich that satisfies those barbecue cravings.

NUTRITIONAL VALUES (PER SERVING):

Calories: 250; Protein: 18g; Carbohydrates: 25g; Fiber: 2g; Total Fat: 8g

Shrimp Pad Thai

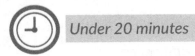 *Under 20 minutes*

INGREDIENTS:

» ½ cup cooked rice noodles
» ¼ cup shrimp, peeled and deveined
» 1 tablespoon Pad Thai sauce

INSTRUCTIONS:

1. In a skillet, with the shrimp pink, which takes about 3-4 minutes, remove from the heat.
2. These ingredients, namely cooked noodles and Pad Thai sauce, should be tossed together.
3. Chopped peanuts (or green onions) may be used if desired and should be served warm. This quick shrimp Pad Thai is delicious, fast, and easy, which makes it an ideal Asian dish for lunch/dinner.

NUTRITIONAL VALUES (PER SERVING):

Calories: 240; Protein: 12g; Carbohydrates: 35g; Fiber: 2g; Total Fat: 6g

Spaghetti with Pesto

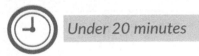 *Under 20 minutes*

INGREDIENTS:

» 1 cup cooked spaghetti
» 2 tablespoons pesto sauce
» Parmesan cheese for garnish

INSTRUCTIONS:

1. Coat cooked spaghetti equally with pesto sauce by tossing it in a big bowl.
2. Serve warm, garnished with Parmesan cheese if desired.
3. This spaghetti with pesto is fresh and vibrant, offering an easy Italian-inspired meal that's both satisfying and quick to prepare.

NUTRITIONAL VALUES (PER SERVING):

Calories: 280; Protein: 8g; Carbohydrates: 42g; Fiber: 2g; Total Fat: 10g

Baked Ziti

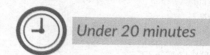

Under 20 minutes

INGREDIENTS:

» 1 cup cooked ziti pasta
» ¼ cup marinara sauce
» ¼ cup mozzarella cheese, shredded

INSTRUCTIONS:

1. Preheat oven to 375°F. In a baking dish, combine cooked ziti and marinara sauce, then sprinkle with mozzarella cheese.
2. Bake for 10 minutes until cheese is melted and bubbly.
3. Warm up before serving. This baked ziti is cheesy and warm, making it a flavorful and easy Italian-style dinner.

NUTRITIONAL VALUES (PER SERVING):

Calories: 300; Protein: 12g; Carbohydrates: 40g; Fiber: 3g; Total Fat: 10g

Greek Chicken Kabobs

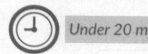

Under 20 minutes

INGREDIENTS:

» ½ cup diced chicken breast
» ¼ cup bell peppers, diced
» 1 tablespoon olive oil
» 1 teaspoon Greek seasoning

INSTRUCTIONS:

1. Thread chicken and bell peppers onto skewers, then brush with olive oil and sprinkle with Greek seasoning.
2. Grill for 5-7 minutes, turning occasionally, until chicken is cooked through.
3. Serve immediately. These Greek chicken kabobs are flavorful and easy, perfect for a quick, Mediterranean-inspired meal.

NUTRITIONAL VALUES (PER SERVING):

Calories: 200; Protein: 18g; Carbohydrates: 4g; Fiber: 1g; Total Fat: 12g

Vegan Lentil Curry

 Under 20 minutes

INGREDIENTS:

» ½ cup cooked lentils
» ¼ cup coconut milk
» 1 teaspoon curry powder

INSTRUCTIONS:

1. Put lentils, coconut milk, and curry powder into a saucepan and continue to simmer on medium heat for about 5-7 minutes.
2. Seeds are enjoyed hot with rice or any Indian bread such as naan. This lentil curry recipe is quick to prepare, has a lot of flavor, and is a great way to deliver healthy vegan protein at any time of day.

NUTRITIONAL VALUES (PER SERVING):

Calories: 180; Protein: 8g; Carbohydrates: 22g; Fiber: 6g; Total Fat: 6g

Chicken Tortilla Soup

 Under 20 minutes

INGREDIENTS:

» 1 cup chicken broth
» ½ cup cooked chicken, shredded
» ¼ cup diced tomatoes
» Tortilla chips for garnish

INSTRUCTIONS:

1. In a pot, place chicken broth, cooked and shredded chicken, and diced tomatoes and allow it to cook for 10 minutes.
2. Served hot and sprinkled with tortilla chips and recommended accompaniments that include avocado or cheese. This chicken tortilla soup is hot filling and is an absolutely perfect fit for a quick bite, rapid lunch, or whatever meal's in a rush.

NUTRITIONAL VALUES (PER SERVING):

Calories: 150; Protein: 10g; Carbohydrates: 12g; Fiber: 2g; Total Fat: 6g

Turkey Chili

 Under 20 minutes

INGREDIENTS:

» ½ cup ground turkey, cooked
» ½ cup kidney beans
» ¼ cup diced tomatoes
» 1 teaspoon chilli powder

INSTRUCTIONS:

1. Blend ground turkey, kidney beans, diced tomatoes, and chili powder in a pot. Cook for 10-15 minutes.
2. They want them hot, so get them hot, then garnish them with some sour cream or shredded cheese or anything. Rich, spicy, and with a comforting without fuss, high protein supper that can be thrown together if you want to slow up.

NUTRITIONAL VALUES (PER SERVING):

Calories: 220; Protein: 15g; Carbohydrates: 20g; Fiber: 6g; Total Fat: 8g

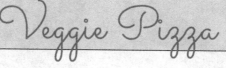

Veggie Pizza

 Under 20 minutes

INGREDIENTS:

» 1 small pizza crust
» ¼ cup marinara sauce
» ¼ cup mixed veggies (bell peppers, olives, mushrooms)
» ¼ cup shredded mozzarella cheese

INSTRUCTIONS:

1. Preheat oven to 400°F. Spread marinara sauce over the pizza crust, then top with mixed veggies and mozzarella.
2. Bake for 10-12 minutes until cheese is melted and bubbly.
3. Serve hot. This veggie pizza is colorful, cheesy, and packed with flavor, making it an easy and satisfying meal.

NUTRITIONAL VALUES (PER SERVING):

Calories: 280; Protein: 10g; Carbohydrates: 36g; Fiber: 4g; Total Fat: 10g

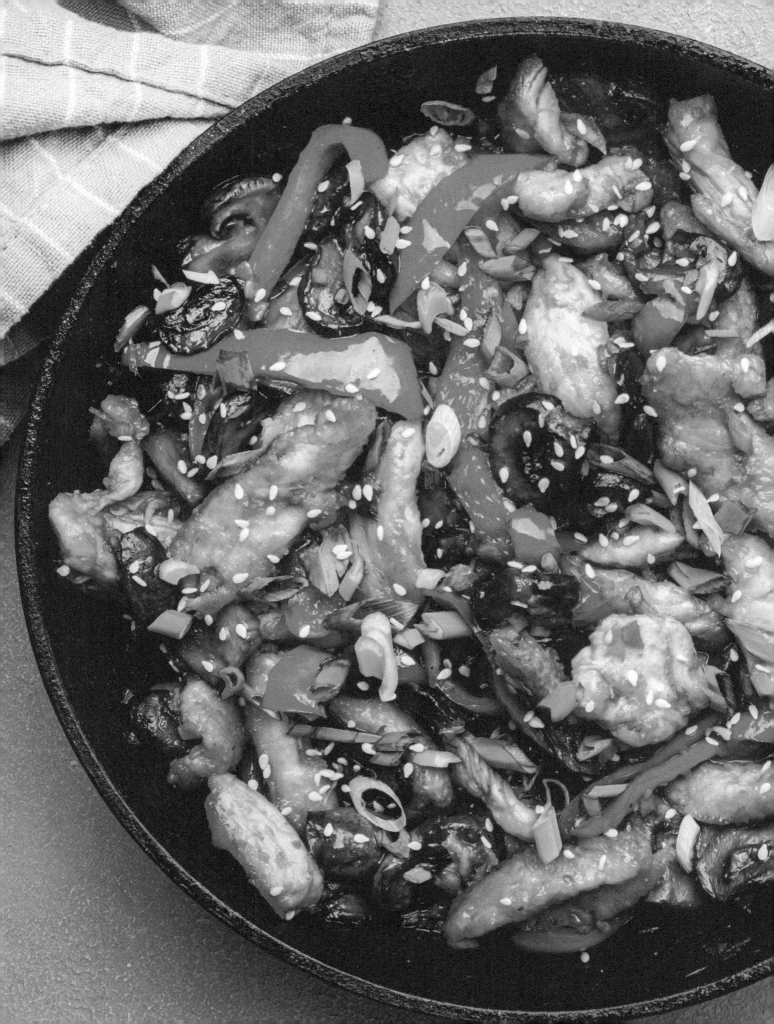

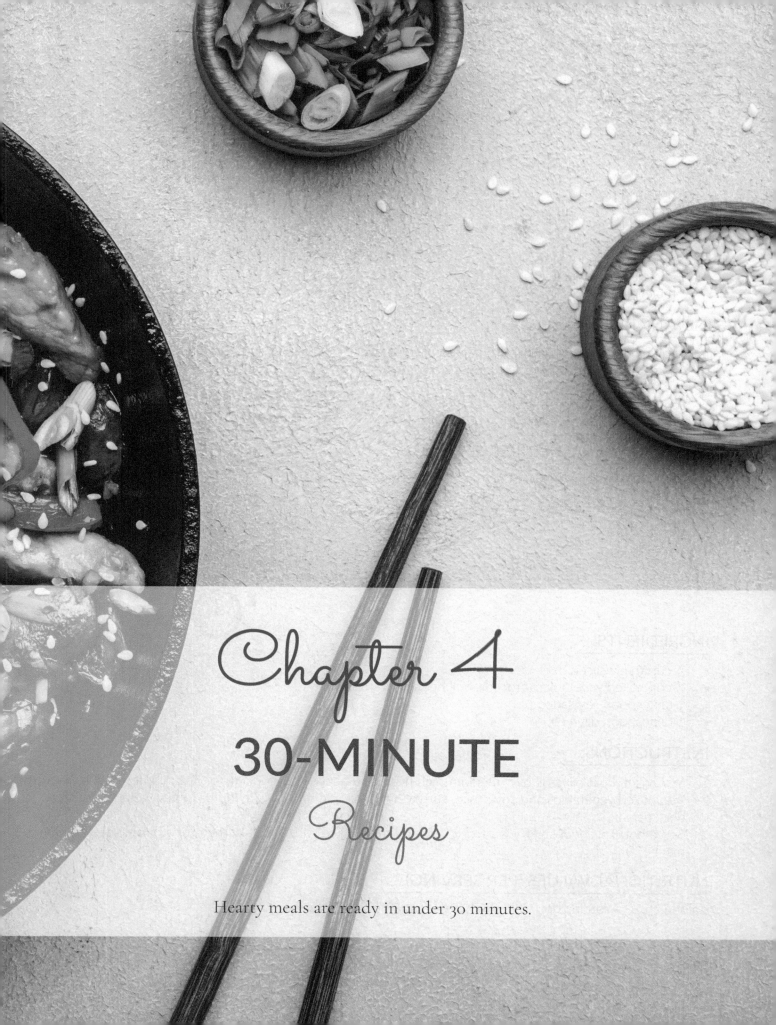

Chapter 4

30-MINUTE

Recipes

Hearty meals are ready in under 30 minutes.

Chicken Cacciatore

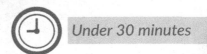 *Under 30 minutes*

INGREDIENTS:

- » 1 chicken breast, diced
- » ½ cup diced tomatoes
- » ¼ cup bell peppers, sliced
- » 1 garlic clove, minced
- » 1 tablespoon olive oil

INSTRUCTIONS:

1. Add the chicken to a skillet with heated olive oil over medium heat and cook until browned.
2. Add garlic, tomatoes, and bell peppers, cooking for an additional 10-12 minutes until the sauce thickens and the chicken is cooked through.
3. Served warm with pasta or rice. If you make this chicken cacciatore in bulk, you can simply freeze the left-over portions for another time, and it makes a hearty and flavor-packed meal in less than 30 minutes.

NUTRITIONAL VALUES (PER SERVING):

Calories: 260; Protein: 22g; Carbohydrates: 8g; Fiber: 2g; Total Fat: 15g

Beef Stir-Fry with Veggies

 Under 30 minutes

INGREDIENTS:

- » ½ cup thinly sliced beef
- » ½ cup mixed vegetables (broccoli, bell peppers, carrots)
- » 1 tablespoon soy sauce
- » 1 tablespoon olive oil

INSTRUCTIONS:

1. In a skillet, heat olive oil over medium-high heat. Add beef slices, cooking for 3-4 minutes until browned.
2. Add mixed vegetables and soy sauce, stir-frying for an additional 5-7 minutes until vegetables are tender-crisp.
3. Serve hot. This beef stir-fry is savory, colorful, and packed with flavor, perfect for a balanced, satisfying meal.

NUTRITIONAL VALUES (PER SERVING):

Calories: 220; Protein: 18g; Carbohydrates: 10g; Fiber: 3g; Total Fat: 12g

Chicken Stir-Fry

 Under 30 minutes

INGREDIENTS:

» 1 chicken breast, diced
» ½ cup bell peppers, sliced
» 1 tablespoon soy sauce
» 1 tablespoon sesame oil

INSTRUCTIONS:

1. In a pan, heat the sesame oil over medium-high heat. Add the chicken and simmer for approximately five minutes or until browned.
2. Add bell peppers and soy sauce, stir-frying for an additional 5-7 minutes until peppers are tender.
3. Serve warm. This chicken stir-fry occurs quickly, produces delicious food, and is great for people who need high-protein meals.

NUTRITIONAL VALUES (PER SERVING):

Calories: 210; Protein: 25g; Carbohydrates: 6g; Fiber: 2g; Total Fat: 10g

Thai Green Curry

 Under 30 minutes

INGREDIENTS:

» ½ cup coconut milk
» ¼ cup green curry paste
» 1 chicken breast, diced
» ½ cup mixed vegetables

INSTRUCTIONS:

1. You place coconut milk in a pan and stir the green curry paste until the mix is even.
2. Simmer chicken and vegetables for 15 minutes; when chicken is cooked and flavors are blended, add chicken and vegetables.
3. Serve warm with rice. This Thai green curry is creamy and spicy with heaps of flavor, which makes it a quick, hearty meal.

NUTRITIONAL VALUES (PER SERVING):

Calories: 280; Protein: 18g; Carbohydrates: 12g; Fiber: 3g; Total Fat: 16g

Cajun Shrimp and Grits

 Under 30 minutes

INGREDIENTS:

» ½ cup shrimp, peeled and deveined
» ¼ cup quick-cooking grits
» 1 teaspoon Cajun seasoning
» 1 tablespoon butter

INSTRUCTIONS:

1. Cook grits according to package instructions. In a skillet, melt butter over medium heat and add shrimp, sprinkling with Cajun seasoning.
2. Sauté shrimp for 3-4 minutes until pink.
3. Serve shrimp over grits for a comforting, Southern-inspired meal with a kick of spice.

NUTRITIONAL VALUES (PER SERVING):

Calories: 220; Protein: 15g; Carbohydrates: 18g; Fiber: 2g; Total Fat: 10g

Chicken Shawarma

 Under 30 minutes

INGREDIENTS:

» 1 chicken breast, sliced
» 1 teaspoon shawarma seasoning
» 1 tablespoon olive oil
» 1 pita bread

INSTRUCTIONS:

1. In a skillet over medium heat, warm olive oil and add chicken, seasoning with shawarma spices. Cook for 10-12 minutes until fully cooked.
2. If you choose to do so, serve the chicken in pita bread with lettuce, tomatoes, and yogurt sauce. This chicken shawarma is loaded with Middle Eastern flavors, so it's a fast and flavorful meal.

NUTRITIONAL VALUES (PER SERVING):

Calories: 300; Protein: 22g; Carbohydrates: 26g; Fiber: 3g; Total Fat: 12g

Pork Stir-Fry with Peppers

 Under 30 minutes

INGREDIENTS:

- » ½ cup pork tenderloin, sliced
- » ½ cup bell peppers, sliced
- » 1 tablespoon soy sauce
- » 1 tablespoon vegetable oil

INSTRUCTIONS:

1. In a skillet, heat vegetable oil over medium-high heat. Add pork, cooking until browned, about 5 minutes.
2. Add bell peppers and soy sauce, stir-frying for another 5-7 minutes until tender-crisp.
3. Serve warm. This pork stir-fry is a quick, savory meal with vibrant bell peppers for a balanced dinner.

NUTRITIONAL VALUES (PER SERVING):

Calories: 220; Protein: 20g; Carbohydrates: 8g; Fiber: 2g; Total Fat: 12g

Stuffed Zucchini

 Under 30 minutes

INGREDIENTS:

- » 1 zucchini, halved and scooped
- » ¼ cup ground turkey, cooked
- » 2 tablespoons marinara sauce
- » 2 tablespoons shredded mozzarella

INSTRUCTIONS:

1. Preheat oven to 375°F. Stuff each zucchini half with ground turkey and marinara sauce, then sprinkle with mozzarella.
2. Bake for 12-15 minutes until cheese is melted and bubbly.
3. Serve warm. This stuffed zucchini is light, tasty, and packed with flavors, making it a healthy and hearty meal.

NUTRITIONAL VALUES (PER SERVING):

Calories: 180; Protein: 15g; Carbohydrates: 6g; Fiber: 2g; Total Fat: 10g

Vegetarian Shepherd's Pie

 Under 30 minutes

INGREDIENTS:

- » ½ cup mixed vegetables (peas, carrots, corn)
- » ¼ cup lentils, cooked
- » ½ cup mashed potatoes

INSTRUCTIONS:

1. In a small baking dish, vegetable and lentil mixture goes in. Mash the boiled potatoes and apply layer over layer on the top as crust.
2. Bake at 375°F for 15-20 minutes until the potatoes are golden and the filling is warm.
3. Serve immediately. Hearty, comforting, and filled with flavors, this vegetarian shepherd's pie is the ideal quick meatless meal.

NUTRITIONAL VALUES (PER SERVING):

Calories: 220; Protein: 8g; Carbohydrates: 36g; Fiber: 5g; Total Fat: 5g

Beef Tacos with Avocado Salsa

 Under 30 minutes

INGREDIENTS:

- » ½ cup ground beef, cooked
- » 2 small tortillas
- » ¼ avocado, diced
- » 1 tablespoon diced tomato

INSTRUCTIONS:

1. Fill each tortilla with cooked ground beef.
2. In a small bowl, combine avocado and tomato for salsa, then spoon over the beef.
3. Serve immediately. These beef tacos with avocado salsa are fresh, flavorful, and perfect for a quick, satisfying meal with a Mexican flair.

NUTRITIONAL VALUES (PER SERVING):

Calories: 280; Protein: 15g; Carbohydrates: 22g; Fiber: 4g; Total Fat: 16g

Grilled Chicken with Garlic Butter

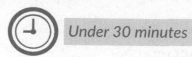 *Under 30 minutes*

INGREDIENTS:

» 1 chicken breast
» 1 tablespoon butter, melted
» 1 garlic clove, minced
» Salt and pepper to taste

INSTRUCTIONS:

1. Preheat a grill or skillet over medium heat. Season chicken breast with salt and pepper.
2. Cook on a grill for 6–7 minutes on each side. Brush with the melted butter and minced garlic in the final minute of frying.
3. Hot from the pot. For a quick and filling dinner, this grilled chicken with garlic butter is succulent, juicy, and bursting with flavor.

NUTRITIONAL VALUES (PER SERVING):

Calories: 220; Protein: 24g; Carbohydrates: 1g; Fiber: 0g; Total Fat: 12g

Pork Tenderloin with Potatoes

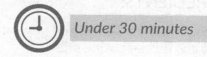 *Under 30 minutes*

INGREDIENTS:

» 1 pork tenderloin, sliced
» ½ cup baby potatoes, halved
» 1 tablespoon olive oil
» Salt, pepper, and rosemary to taste

INSTRUCTIONS:

1. Preheat oven to 400°F. Toss potatoes with olive oil, salt, pepper, and rosemary. Arrange on a baking sheet with pork slices.
2. Bake for 20-25 minutes until pork is cooked and potatoes are tender.
3. Serve immediately. This pork tenderloin with potatoes recipe is easy, delicious, and can be made quickly for that satisfying dinner.

NUTRITIONAL VALUES (PER SERVING):

Calories: 260; Protein: 22g; Carbohydrates: 15g; Fiber: 2g; Total Fat: 10g

Bbq Beef Ribs

 Under 30 minutes

INGREDIENTS:

» ½ pound beef ribs
» ¼ cup BBQ sauce
» Salt and pepper to taste

INSTRUCTIONS:

1. Preheat oven to 375°F. Season ribs with salt and pepper, then brush with BBQ sauce.
2. Bake for 25-30 minutes, turning halfway through and basting with extra sauce.
3. Serve hot. Tender, smokey, and brimming with flavor, these BBQ beef ribs make a quick yet filling dinner.

NUTRITIONAL VALUES (PER SERVING):

Calories: 400; Protein: 22g; Carbohydrates: 8g; Fiber: 1g; Total Fat: 30g

Shrimp and Grits

 Under 30 minutes

INGREDIENTS:

» ½ cup shrimp, peeled and deveined
» ¼ cup quick-cooking grits
» 1 tablespoon butter
» 1 teaspoon Cajun seasoning

INSTRUCTIONS:

1. Grits should then be boiled according to the directions on the pack. In the skillet, melt the butter, add the shrimp, and add the Cajun spice.
2. Cook shrimp until pink in color, approximately 3-4 minutes.
3. Offer shrimp over grits as an easy Southern-style dish. It is rich in texture, hot in texture, and hot in flavor.

NUTRITIONAL VALUES (PER SERVING):

Calories: 220; Protein: 15g; Carbohydrates: 20g; Fiber: 2g; Total Fat: 10g

Salmon with Dill Cream

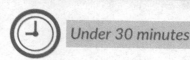 *Under 30 minutes*

INGREDIENTS:

- » 1 salmon fillet
- » 1 tablespoon sour cream
- » 1 teaspoon fresh dill, chopped
- » Lemon wedge for garnish

INSTRUCTIONS:

1. Grill or bake the salmon fillet at 400°F for 12-15 minutes until it flakes easily.
2. In a small bowl, mix sour cream and dill. Spoon over the salmon and serve with a lemon wedge.
3. This salmon with dill cream is light, creamy, and ideal for a quick, healthy meal with fresh flavors.

NUTRITIONAL VALUES (PER SERVING):

Calories: 240; Protein: 22g; Carbohydrates: 1g; Fiber: 0g; Total Fat: 16g

Spicy Chicken Wings

 Under 30 minutes

INGREDIENTS:

- » 6 chicken wings
- » 2 tablespoons hot sauce
- » 1 tablespoon melted butter

INSTRUCTIONS:

1. Preheat oven to 400°F. Toss wings in hot sauce and melted butter until coated.
2. Arrange on a baking sheet and bake for 20-25 minutes until crispy.
3. Serve immediately. These spicy chicken wings are tangy and bold, perfect for a quick snack or appetizer with a spicy kick.

NUTRITIONAL VALUES (PER SERVING):

Calories: 280; Protein: 18g; Carbohydrates: 1g; Fiber: 0g; Total Fat: 22g

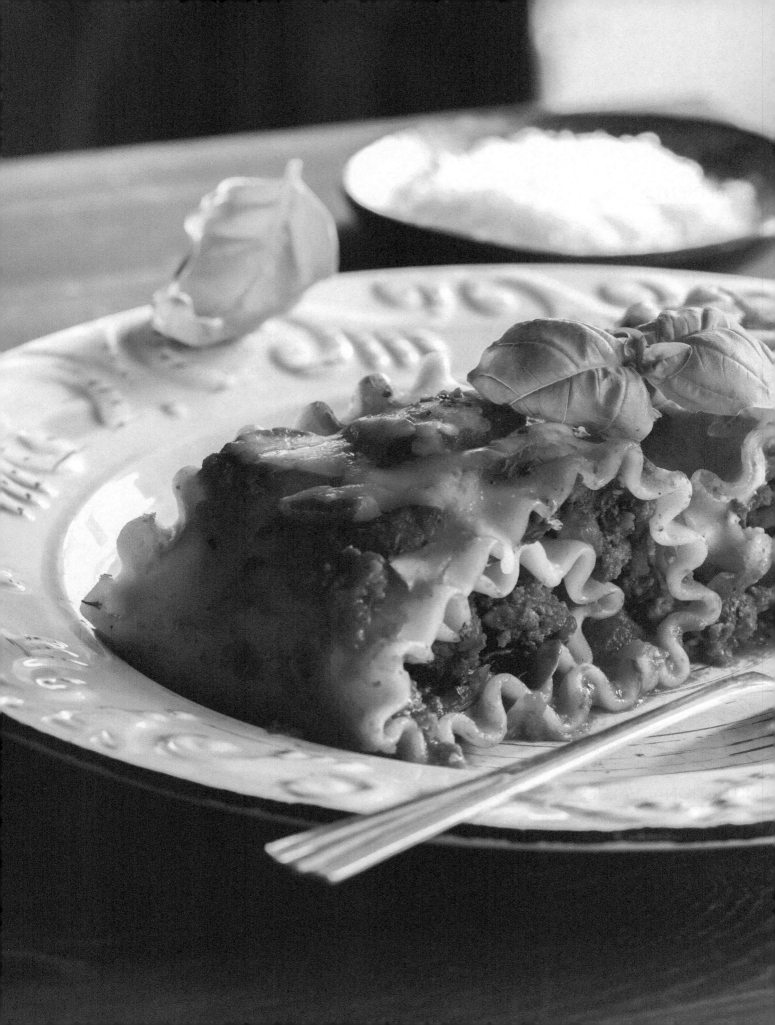

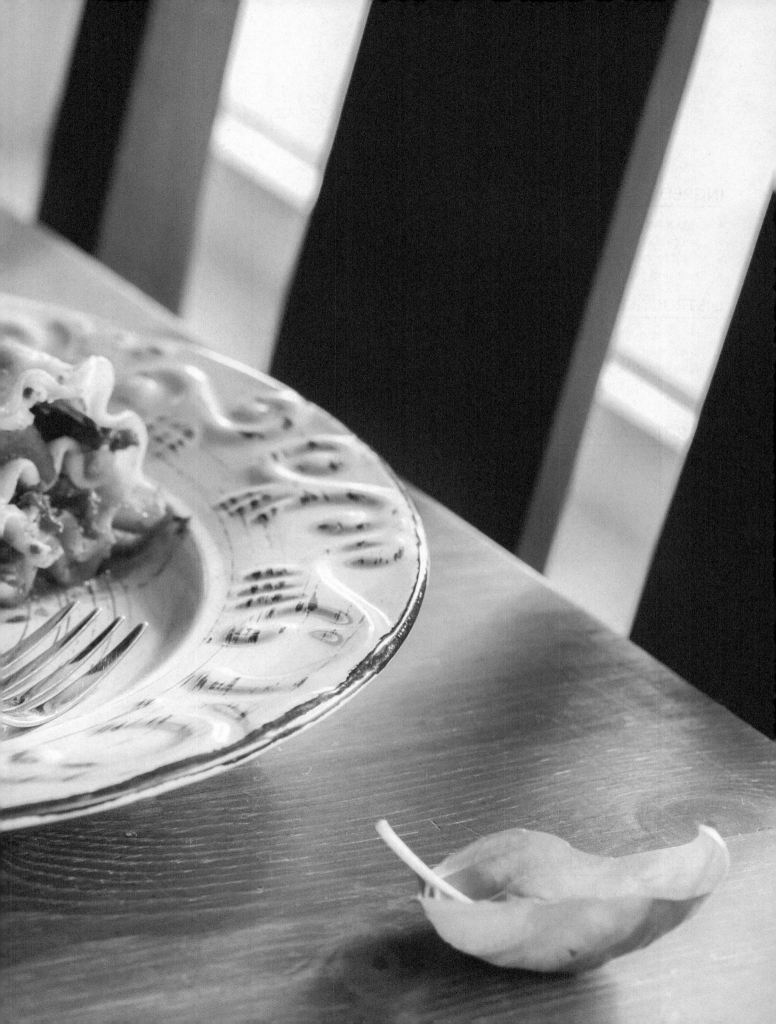

Turkey Meatloaf

 Under 30 minutes

INGREDIENTS:

» ½ pound ground turkey
» ¼ cup breadcrumbs
» 1 tablespoon ketchup
» Salt and pepper to taste

INSTRUCTIONS:

1. Preheat oven to 375°F. In a bowl, mix ground turkey, breadcrumbs, ketchup, salt, and pepper. Shape into a small loaf.
2. Bake for 20-25 minutes until cooked through.
3. Serve hot. This turkey meatloaf is flavorful, moist, and perfect for a comforting, protein-rich meal in no time.

NUTRITIONAL VALUES (PER SERVING):

Calories: 180; Protein: 20g; Carbohydrates: 10g; Fiber: 1g; Total Fat: 8g

Spinach Lasagna Rolls

 Under 30 minutes

INGREDIENTS:

» 2 lasagna noodles, cooked
» ¼ cup ricotta cheese
» ½ cup spinach, chopped
» ¼ cup marinara sauce

INSTRUCTIONS:

1. Preheat oven to 375°F. Spread ricotta and spinach over each noodle, then roll up. Place in a baking dish and cover with marinara sauce.
2. Bake for 15-20 minutes until heated through.
3. Serve warm. These spinach lasagna rolls are cheesy, flavorful, and a great vegetarian option for a quick Italian-inspired meal.

NUTRITIONAL VALUES (PER SERVING):

Calories: 200; Protein: 10g; Carbohydrates: 25g; Fiber: 3g; Total Fat: 8g

Chicken Tikka Masala

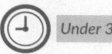 *Under 30 minutes*

INGREDIENTS:

» 1 chicken breast, cubed
» ¼ cup tikka masala sauce
» 1 tablespoon olive oil

INSTRUCTIONS:

1. In a skillet over medium heat, warm olive oil and cook chicken until browned.
2. Add tikka masala sauce, stirring to coat, and simmer for 10-12 minutes until chicken is cooked through.
3. Serve with rice or naan. This chicken tikka masala is rich flavorful, and offers a quick, satisfying Indian-inspired meal.

NUTRITIONAL VALUES (PER SERVING):

Calories: 240; Protein: 24g; Carbohydrates: 6g; Fiber: 1g; Total Fat: 14g

Beef and Bean Burritos

 Under 30 minutes

INGREDIENTS:

» ½ cup ground beef, cooked
» ¼ cup black beans
» 1 large tortilla
» 1 tablespoon salsa

INSTRUCTIONS:

1. Put the ground beef and black beans on the midsection of the tortilla.
2. Place a spoonful of salsa over the filling and then regard the end of the tortilla and fold it till it is well covered.
3. It said it needs to be served warm and can be garnished with sour cream. This burrito recipe is packed with seasoned ground beef and beans, making it a fantastic quick Mexican dinner.

NUTRITIONAL VALUES (PER SERVING):

Calories: 320; Protein: 16g; Carbohydrates: 30g; Fiber: 4g; Total Fat: 14g

Vegetable Stir-Fry with Tofu

 Under 30 minutes

INGREDIENTS:

» ½ cup tofu, cubed
» 1 cup mixed vegetables (broccoli, bell peppers, carrots)
» 1 tablespoon soy sauce
» 1 tablespoon olive oil

INSTRUCTIONS:

1. In a skillet, heat olive oil over medium heat. Add tofu cubes and cook until golden, about 5 minutes.
2. Add mixed vegetables and soy sauce, stir-frying for 5-7 minutes until tender-crisp.
3. Serve warm. This vegetable stir fry with tofu is really rich in colors; it makes a healthy and easy option for vegetarian cooks.

NUTRITIONAL VALUES (PER SERVING):

Calories: 200; Protein: 10g; Carbohydrates: 12g; Fiber: 3g; Total Fat: 12g

Roasted Chicken with Root Vegetables

 Under 30 minutes

INGREDIENTS:

» 1 chicken thigh
» ½ cup root vegetables (carrots, potatoes), diced
» 1 tablespoon olive oil
» Salt, pepper, and rosemary to taste

INSTRUCTIONS:

1. Preheat oven to 400°F. Toss root vegetables with olive oil, salt, pepper, and rosemary.
2. Place chicken and vegetables on a baking sheet and roast for 25 minutes until chicken is cooked and vegetables are tender.
3. Serve warm. This roasted chicken with root vegetables is hearty, flavorful, and ideal for a balanced, home-cooked meal.

NUTRITIONAL VALUES (PER SERVING):

Calories: 260; Protein: 18g; Carbohydrates: 15g; Fiber: 3g; Total Fat: 14g

Italian Sausage and Peppers

 Under 30 minutes

INGREDIENTS:

- » 1 Italian sausage link, sliced
- » ½ cup bell peppers, sliced
- » 1 tablespoon olive oil

INSTRUCTIONS:

1. In a skillet, heat olive oil over medium heat. Add sausage slices and cook until browned.
2. Add bell peppers and cook for an additional 5-7 minutes until peppers are tender.
3. Serve hot. This Italian sausage and peppers dish is savory and colorful and makes for a quick, filling meal full of classic flavors.

NUTRITIONAL VALUES (PER SERVING):

Calories: 250; Protein: 12g; Carbohydrates: 8g; Fiber: 2g; Total Fat: 18g

Spaghetti with Clam Sauce

 Under 30 minutes

INGREDIENTS:

- » 1 cup cooked spaghetti
- » ¼ cup canned clams, drained
- » 1 tablespoon olive oil
- » 1 garlic clove, minced

INSTRUCTIONS:

1. In a skillet, heat olive oil over medium heat. Add garlic and clams, sautéing for 2-3 minutes.
2. Toss with cooked spaghetti and season with salt and pepper.
3. Serve hot, optionally garnished with parsley. This spaghetti with clam sauce is light, briny, and perfect for a quick, seafood-inspired meal.

NUTRITIONAL VALUES (PER SERVING):

Calories: 260; Protein: 10g; Carbohydrates: 42g; Fiber: 2g; Total Fat: 8g

Vegan Mushroom Stroganoff

 Under 30 minutes

INGREDIENTS:

- » 1 cup mushrooms, sliced
- » ½ cup coconut milk
- » 1 tablespoon olive oil
- » 1 teaspoon paprika

INSTRUCTIONS:

1. In a skillet, heat olive oil over medium heat. Add mushrooms and cook until tender.
2. Stir in coconut milk and paprika, simmering for 5-7 minutes.
3. Serve over rice or pasta. This vegan mushroom stroganoff is creamy, flavorful, and ideal for a quick, satisfying plant-based meal.

NUTRITIONAL VALUES (PER SERVING):

Calories: 180; Protein: 4g; Carbohydrates: 8g; Fiber: 2g; Total Fat: 14g

Grilled Pork Chops with Apples

 Under 30 minutes

INGREDIENTS:

- » 1 pork chop
- » ½ apple, sliced
- » 1 tablespoon olive oil
- » 1 teaspoon honey

INSTRUCTIONS:

1. Heat olive oil in a skillet over medium heat. Cook pork chop for 5-6 minutes per side until browned and cooked through.
2. Add apple slices and drizzle with honey, cooking for another 2-3 minutes.
3. Serve hot. These grilled pork chops with apples are sweet and savory, perfect for a comforting meal.

NUTRITIONAL VALUES (PER SERVING):

Calories: 280; Protein: 22g; Carbohydrates: 10g; Fiber: 2g; Total Fat: 16g

Black Bean Enchiladas

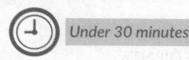 *Under 30 minutes*

INGREDIENTS:

» 2 corn tortillas
» ½ cup black beans
» ¼ cup enchilada sauce
» 2 tablespoons shredded cheese

INSTRUCTIONS:

1. Preheat oven to 375°F. Fill each tortilla with black beans and a little enchilada sauce, then roll it up and place it in a baking dish.
2. Cover with more enchilada sauce and sprinkle with cheese.
3. Bake for 15-20 minutes until cheese is melted. These black bean enchiladas are hearty, cheesy, and perfect for a quick, vegetarian, Mexican-inspired meal.

NUTRITIONAL VALUES (PER SERVING):

Calories: 240; Protein: 10g; Carbohydrates: 30g; Fiber: 6g; Total Fat: 8g

Shrimp Gumbo

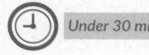 *Under 30 minutes*

INGREDIENTS:

» ½ cup shrimp, peeled and deveined
» ½ cup okra, sliced
» ¼ cup diced tomatoes
» 1 cup chicken broth

INSTRUCTIONS:

1. In a pot, combine shrimp, okra, tomatoes, and chicken broth. Bring to a simmer and cook for 15-20 minutes until flavors meld and shrimp is cooked through.
2. Serve hot. This shrimp gumbo is spicy, flavorful, and ideal for a quick taste of the South.

NUTRITIONAL VALUES (PER SERVING):

Calories: 180; Protein: 14g; Carbohydrates: 8g; Fiber: 2g; Total Fat: 8g

Teriyaki Chicken Skewers

 Under 30 minutes

INGREDIENTS:

- » 1 chicken breast, cubed
- » 2 tablespoons teriyaki sauce
- » Bell pepper and pineapple chunks

INSTRUCTIONS:

1. Thread chicken, bell pepper, and pineapple onto skewers, then brush with teriyaki sauce.
2. Grill over medium heat for 10-12 minutes, turning and basting with extra sauce.
3. Serve hot. These teriyaki chicken skewers are sweet, savory, and perfect for a quick meal with tropical flavors.

NUTRITIONAL VALUES (PER SERVING):

Calories: 250; Protein: 20g; Carbohydrates: 12g; Fiber: 2g; Total Fat: 10g

Chicken Alfredo Pasta Bake

 Under 30 minutes

INGREDIENTS:

- » 1 cup cooked pasta
- » ½ cup cooked chicken, diced
- » ¼ cup Alfredo sauce
- » 2 tablespoons mozzarella cheese

INSTRUCTIONS:

1. Preheat oven to 375°F. In a baking dish, mix pasta, chicken, and Alfredo sauce, then sprinkle with mozzarella.
2. Bake for 15-20 minutes until cheese is melted and bubbly.
3. Serve hot. This method creates a creamy bake and is definitely ideal for a quick Italian dinner of chicken Alfredo pasta.

NUTRITIONAL VALUES (PER SERVING):

Calories: 300; Protein: 18g; Carbohydrates: 30g; Fiber: 2g; Total Fat: 12g

Baked Falafel with Tzatziki

 Under 30 minutes

INGREDIENTS:

» ½ cup canned chickpeas, drained
» 1 tablespoon parsley, chopped
» 1 garlic clove, minced
» 2 tablespoons tzatziki sauce

INSTRUCTIONS:

1. Preheat oven to 400°F. Let the chickpeas, parsley, and garlic be mashed and shaped into small round discs.
2. Spread on a baking tray and bake for about twenty minutes until brown and crispy.
3. Serve with tzatziki sauce. This baked falafel with tzatziki is crispy on the outside and loaded with Mediterranean flavor, which is perfect for a quick, healthy snack or meal.

NUTRITIONAL VALUES (PER SERVING):

Calories: 180; Protein: 7g; Carbohydrates: 20g; Fiber: 5g; Total Fat: 8g

Lamb Curry with Rice

 Under 30 minutes

INGREDIENTS:

» ½ cup lamb, diced
» ¼ cup coconut milk
» 1 teaspoon curry powder
» 1 cup cooked rice

INSTRUCTIONS:

1. In a skillet, sauté the lamb on medium heat until it is done to a brownish color. Pour curry powder and coconut milk and let it boil for another 15 minutes.
2. Serve hot cooked rice. A delicious and warming curry with simple ingredients and flavored rice, this lamb curry can be on the table quickly.

NUTRITIONAL VALUES (PER SERVING):

Calories: 300; Protein: 18g; Carbohydrates: 32g; Fiber: 2g; Total Fat: 12g

Chili Mac and Cheese

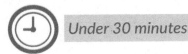 *Under 30 minutes*

INGREDIENTS:

» ½ cup cooked macaroni
» ¼ cup ground beef
» ¼ cup shredded cheddar cheese
» 2 tablespoons salsa

INSTRUCTIONS:

1. In a skillet, cook ground beef until browned. Add salsa and cooked macaroni, stirring until combined.
2. Sprinkle cheddar cheese on top and let it melt for a minute.
3. Serve warm. This chili mac and cheese is hearty, cheesy, and perfect for a quick, satisfying meal with a spicy twist.

NUTRITIONAL VALUES (PER SERVING):

Calories: 320; Protein: 18g; Carbohydrates: 28g; Fiber: 3g; Total Fat: 16g

Creamy Pesto Chicken

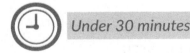 *Under 30 minutes*

INGREDIENTS:

» 1 chicken breast, diced
» 2 tablespoons pesto sauce
» ¼ cup heavy cream

INSTRUCTIONS:

1. In a skillet over medium heat, cook chicken until browned, about 5-7 minutes.
2. Add pesto sauce and cream, stirring until chicken is well coated and sauce is heated through.
3. Serve hot. This creamy pesto chicken is rich, flavorful, and perfect for a quick, comforting meal with Italian-inspired flavors.

NUTRITIONAL VALUES (PER SERVING):

Calories: 280; Protein: 24g; Carbohydrates: 2g; Fiber: 0g; Total Fat: 20g

Moroccan Vegetable Stew

 Under 30 minutes

INGREDIENTS:

» ½ cup chickpeas
» ¼ cup carrots, diced
» ¼ cup zucchini, diced
» 1 teaspoon cumin

INSTRUCTIONS:

1. In a pot, combine chickpeas, carrots, zucchini, and cumin. Add water to cover and bring to a simmer.
2. Cook for 15-20 minutes until vegetables are tender.
3. Serve hot. This Moroccan vegetable stew is spiced and hearty, ideal for a quick, plant-based meal that's both healthy and filling.

NUTRITIONAL VALUES (PER SERVING):

Calories: 180; Protein: 6g; Carbohydrates: 30g; Fiber: 7g; Total Fat: 4g

Beef Stroganoff

 Under 30 minutes

INGREDIENTS:

» ½ cup ground beef
» ¼ cup mushrooms, sliced
» ¼ cup sour cream
» 1 tablespoon olive oil

INSTRUCTIONS:

1. In a skillet over medium heat, cook ground beef and mushrooms until browned.
2. Stir in sour cream, simmering for 5-7 minutes until well combined.
3. Serve over rice or pasta. This beef stroganoff is creamy, rich, and perfect for a comforting, quick meal.

NUTRITIONAL VALUES (PER SERVING):

Calories: 250; Protein: 15g; Carbohydrates: 8g; Fiber: 1g; Total Fat: 18g

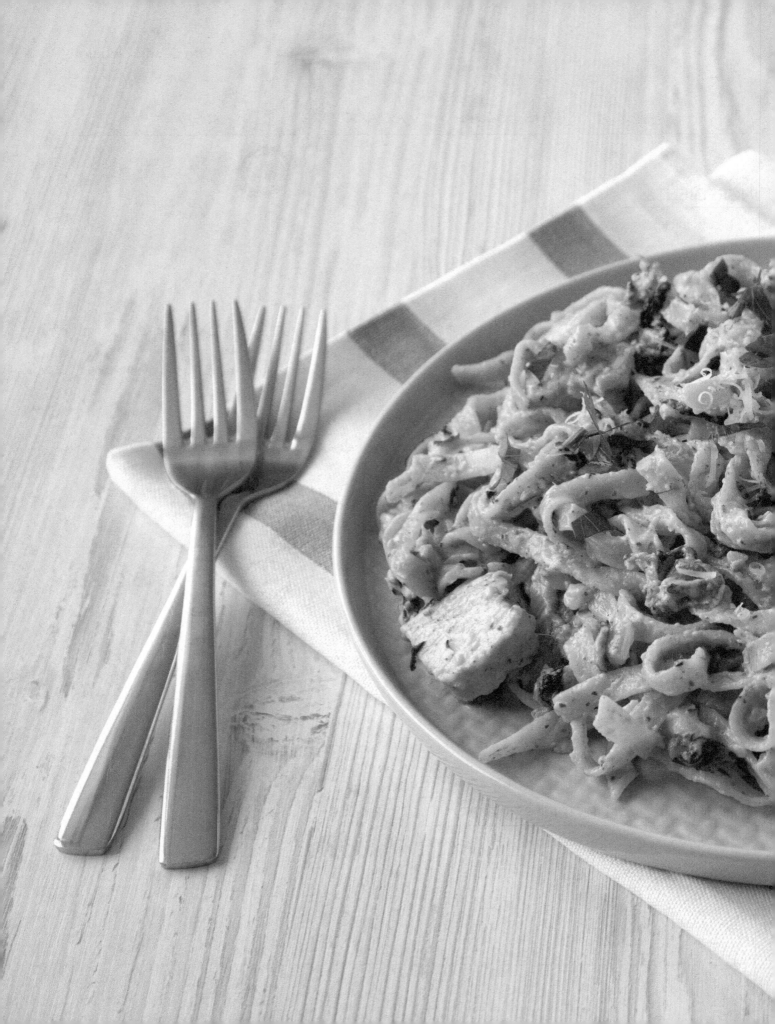

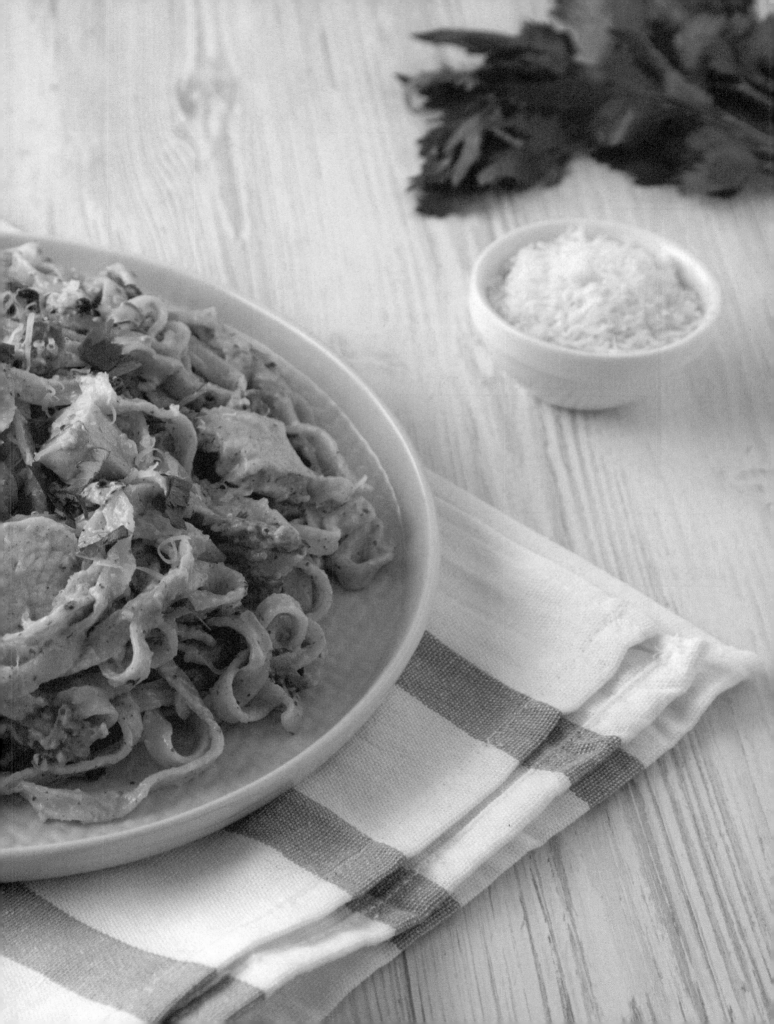

Baked Salmon with Dijon Mustard

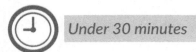 *Under 30 minutes*

INGREDIENTS:

» 1 salmon fillet
» 1 tablespoon Dijon mustard
» 1 teaspoon honey

INSTRUCTIONS:

1. Preheat oven to 400°F. Brush the salmon fillet with Dijon mustard and honey.
2. Bake for 12-15 minutes until the salmon flakes easily with a fork.
3. Serve hot. This baked salmon with Dijon mustard is tangy, sweet, and perfect for a quick, elegant dinner.

NUTRITIONAL VALUES (PER SERVING):

Calories: 230; Protein: 22g; Carbohydrates: 3g; Fiber: 0g; Total Fat: 14g

Bbq Chicken Sandwiches

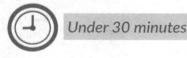 *Under 30 minutes*

INGREDIENTS:

» ½ cup shredded cooked chicken
» 2 tablespoons BBQ sauce
» 1 sandwich roll

INSTRUCTIONS:

1. In a skillet, heat shredded chicken and BBQ sauce until warm and evenly coated.
2. Serve in a sandwich roll, optionally topped with coleslaw.
3. This BBQ chicken sandwich is smoky, tangy, and perfect for a quick, hearty meal.

NUTRITIONAL VALUES (PER SERVING):

Calories: 260; Protein: 18g; Carbohydrates: 32g; Fiber: 2g; Total Fat: 8g

Roasted Brussels Sprouts with Balsamic

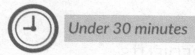 *Under 30 minutes*

INGREDIENTS:

» 1 cup Brussels sprouts, halved
» 1 tablespoon olive oil
» 1 teaspoon balsamic vinegar

INSTRUCTIONS:

1. Preheat oven to 400°F. Toss Brussels sprouts with olive oil and roast for 20 minutes until tender and slightly crispy.
2. Drizzle with balsamic vinegar and serve hot.
3. These roasted Brussels sprouts are savory, tangy, and perfect as a side dish or a light meal.

NUTRITIONAL VALUES (PER SERVING):

Calories: 120; Protein: 4g; Carbohydrates: 12g; Fiber: 5g; Total Fat: 7g

Chicken Fettuccine Alfredo

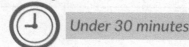 *Under 30 minutes*

INGREDIENTS:

» 1 cup cooked fettuccine
» ½ cup cooked chicken, sliced
» ¼ cup Alfredo sauce

INSTRUCTIONS:

1. In a saucepan, combine fettuccine, chicken, and Alfredo sauce over medium heat, stirring until heated through.
2. Serve warm with Parmesan cheese if desired.
3. This chicken fettuccine Alfredo is creamy, rich, and comforting, perfect for a quick Italian-inspired dinner.

NUTRITIONAL VALUES (PER SERVING):

Calories: 320; Protein: 18g; Carbohydrates: 38g; Fiber: 2g; Total Fat: 12g

Stuffed Bell Peppers

 Under 30 minutes

INGREDIENTS:

» 2 bell peppers, halved and deseeded
» ½ cup ground beef, cooked
» ¼ cup cooked rice
» 2 tablespoons marinara sauce

INSTRUCTIONS:

1. Preheat oven to 375°F. In a bowl, mix ground beef, rice, and marinara sauce.
2. Fill each pepper half with the mixture and place in a baking dish.
3. Bake for 15-20 minutes until peppers are tender. Serve hot. These stuffed bell peppers are savory and nutritious, making for a balanced meal with vibrant flavors.

NUTRITIONAL VALUES (PER SERVING):

Calories: 250; Protein: 12g; Carbohydrates: 28g; Fiber: 5g; Total Fat: 10g

Chicken and Rice Casserole

 Under 30 minutes

INGREDIENTS:

» ½ cup cooked chicken, shredded
» ½ cup cooked rice
» ¼ cup cream of mushroom soup
» Salt and pepper to taste

INSTRUCTIONS:

1. Preheat oven to 375°F. In a baking dish, mix chicken, rice, and cream of mushroom soup, seasoning with salt and pepper.
2. Bake for 15-20 minutes until heated through.
3. Serve warm. This chicken and rice casserole is creamy, hearty, and perfect for a comforting, home-cooked meal.

NUTRITIONAL VALUES (PER SERVING):

Calories: 280; Protein: 20g; Carbohydrates: 30g; Fiber: 2g; Total Fat: 10g

Korean Beef Bulgogi

 Under 30 minutes

INGREDIENTS:

» ½ cup thinly sliced beef
» 1 tablespoon soy sauce
» 1 teaspoon sesame oil
» 1 teaspoon sugar

INSTRUCTIONS:

1. In a skillet over medium-high heat, cook beef with soy sauce, sesame oil, and sugar until browned and caramelized, about 5-7 minutes.
2. Serve with rice or lettuce wraps. This Korean beef bulgogi is savory and slightly sweet, making it a quick, flavorful meal with an authentic taste.

NUTRITIONAL VALUES (PER SERVING):

Calories: 220; Protein: 15g; Carbohydrates: 8g; Fiber: 0g; Total Fat: 14g

Roasted Red Pepper Soup

 Under 30 minutes

INGREDIENTS:

» 1 cup roasted red peppers
» ½ cup vegetable broth
» ¼ cup coconut milk

INSTRUCTIONS:

1. In a pot, roast red peppers, add vegetable broth, and simmer for 10 minutes.
2. Then, use an immersion blender to purée until it's smooth, and stir in coconut milk.
3. Serve warm. This creamy, slightly sweet soup is the perfect comforting, quick meal.

NUTRITIONAL VALUES (PER SERVING):

Calories: 150; Protein: 2g; Carbohydrates: 12g; Fiber: 3g; Total Fat: 10g

Grilled Pork Tenderloin

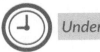 *Under 30 minutes*

INGREDIENTS:

- » 1 pork tenderloin
- » 1 tablespoon olive oil
- » Salt, pepper, and thyme to taste

INSTRUCTIONS:

1. Heat grill on medium-high. Rub olive oil, salt, pepper, and thyme over the pork.
2. Cook thoroughly, turning occasionally, about 12-15 minutes.
3. Slice and serve. And for an incredibly simple, flavorful, easy meal with these few ingredients...this grilled pork tenderloin? TENDER. JUICY. PERFECT.

NUTRITIONAL VALUES (PER SERVING):

Calories: 240; Protein: 24g; Carbohydrates: 0g; Fiber: 0g; Total Fat: 14g

Pasta Primavera

 Under 30 minutes

INGREDIENTS:

- » 1 cup cooked pasta
- » ½ cup mixed vegetables (bell peppers, zucchini, cherry tomatoes)
- » 1 tablespoon olive oil
- » 1 garlic clove, minced

INSTRUCTIONS:

1. In a skillet, heat olive oil over medium heat. Add garlic and mixed vegetables, cooking until tender.
2. Toss with pasta and season with salt and pepper.
3. Serve hot. This pasta primavera is light, fresh, and packed with vegetables, making it a quick, satisfying Italian-inspired meal.

NUTRITIONAL VALUES (PER SERVING):

Calories: 280; Protein: 8g; Carbohydrates: 44g; Fiber: 5g; Total Fat: 10g

Chicken Pho

 Under 30 minutes

INGREDIENTS:

» 1 cup chicken broth
» ½ cup cooked chicken, shredded
» Rice noodles
» Fresh herbs (cilantro, basil) for garnish

INSTRUCTIONS:

1. In a pot, bring chicken broth to a simmer and add cooked chicken and rice noodles, cooking until noodles are soft.
2. Serve in a bowl garnished with fresh herbs. This chicken pho is light, flavorful, and comforting, perfect for a quick Vietnamese-inspired meal.

NUTRITIONAL VALUES (PER SERVING):

Calories: 200; Protein: 15g; Carbohydrates: 30g; Fiber: 2g; Total Fat: 4g

Eggplant Rollatini

 Under 30 minutes

INGREDIENTS:

» 1 small eggplant, thinly sliced
» ¼ cup ricotta cheese
» 2 tablespoons marinara sauce
» 1 tablespoon Parmesan cheese

INSTRUCTIONS:

1. Preheat oven to 375°F. Spread ricotta on each eggplant slice, roll it up, and place it in a baking dish. Top with marinara sauce and Parmesan.
2. Bake for 15-20 minutes until bubbly.
3. Serve warm. This eggplant rollatini is creamy, cheesy, and perfect for a quick, satisfying vegetarian meal.

NUTRITIONAL VALUES (PER SERVING):

Calories: 160; Protein: 6g; Carbohydrates: 12g; Fiber: 4g; Total Fat: 10g

Chicken and Shrimp Paella

 Under 30 minutes

INGREDIENTS:

- » ¼ cup cooked chicken, diced
- » ¼ cup shrimp, peeled
- » ½ cup rice
- » ¼ cup chicken broth

INSTRUCTIONS:

1. In a skillet, combine rice and chicken broth, cooking until rice absorbs the liquid.
2. Add chicken and shrimp, cooking until shrimp is pink and chicken is heated through.
3. Serve warm. This chicken and shrimp paella is flavorful and hearty, bringing Spanish flavors to a quick, filling meal.

NUTRITIONAL VALUES (PER SERVING):

Calories: 300; Protein: 20g; Carbohydrates: 30g; Fiber: 2g; Total Fat: 10g

Bacon-Wrapped Shrimp

 Under 30 minutes

INGREDIENTS:

- » 6 large shrimp, peeled
- » 3 slices bacon, halved
- » 1 teaspoon olive oil

INSTRUCTIONS:

1. Preheat oven to 400°F. Wrap each shrimp with half a slice of bacon and secure with a toothpick.
2. Place on a baking sheet, drizzle with olive oil, and bake for 12-15 minutes until bacon is crispy.
3. Serve warm. These bacon-wrapped shrimp are smoky and savory and make for an easy, elegant appetizer or main dish.

NUTRITIONAL VALUES (PER SERVING):

Calories: 180; Protein: 12g; Carbohydrates: 1g; Fiber: 0g; Total Fat: 14g

Baked Chicken with Lemon Garlic

 Under 30 minutes

INGREDIENTS:

» 1 chicken breast
» 1 tablespoon olive oil
» 1 clove garlic, minced
» 1 tablespoon lemon juice

INSTRUCTIONS:

1. Preheat oven to 375°F. Place chicken breast in a baking dish, drizzle with olive oil, and season with garlic and lemon juice.
2. Bake for 20-25 minutes until the chicken is cooked through and golden.
3. Serve warm. This baked chicken with lemon garlic is flavorful, juicy, and perfect for a quick, satisfying meal that's both light and aromatic.

NUTRITIONAL VALUES (PER SERVING):

Calories: 220; Protein: 24g; Carbohydrates: 1g; Fiber: 0g; Total Fat: 12g

Vegetarian Chili with Sweet Potatoes

 Under 30 minutes

INGREDIENTS:

» ½ cup black beans
» ½ cup diced sweet potatoes
» 1 cup diced tomatoes
» 1 teaspoon chili powder

INSTRUCTIONS:

1. In a pot, combine black beans, sweet potatoes, diced tomatoes, and chili powder.
2. Simmer for 15-20 minutes until sweet potatoes are tender.
3. Serve warm, optionally garnished with sour cream. This vegetarian chili is hearty, filling, and rich in flavor, perfect for a comforting plant-based meal.

NUTRITIONAL VALUES (PER SERVING):

Calories: 180; Protein: 6g; Carbohydrates: 30g; Fiber: 8g; Total Fat: 2g

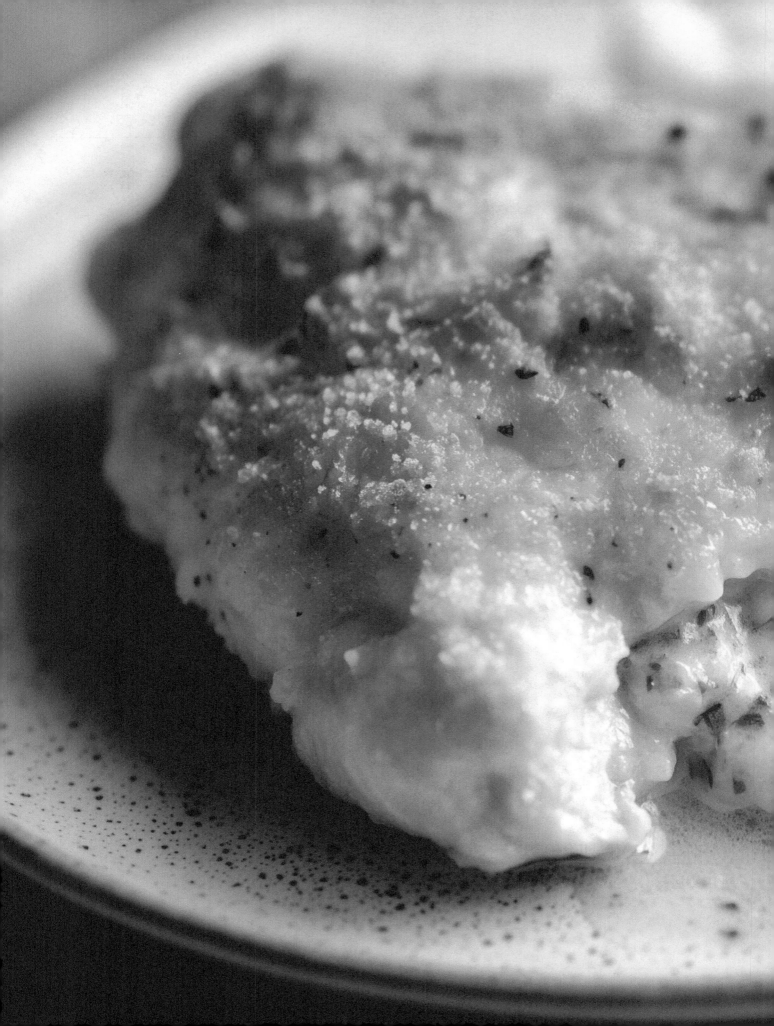

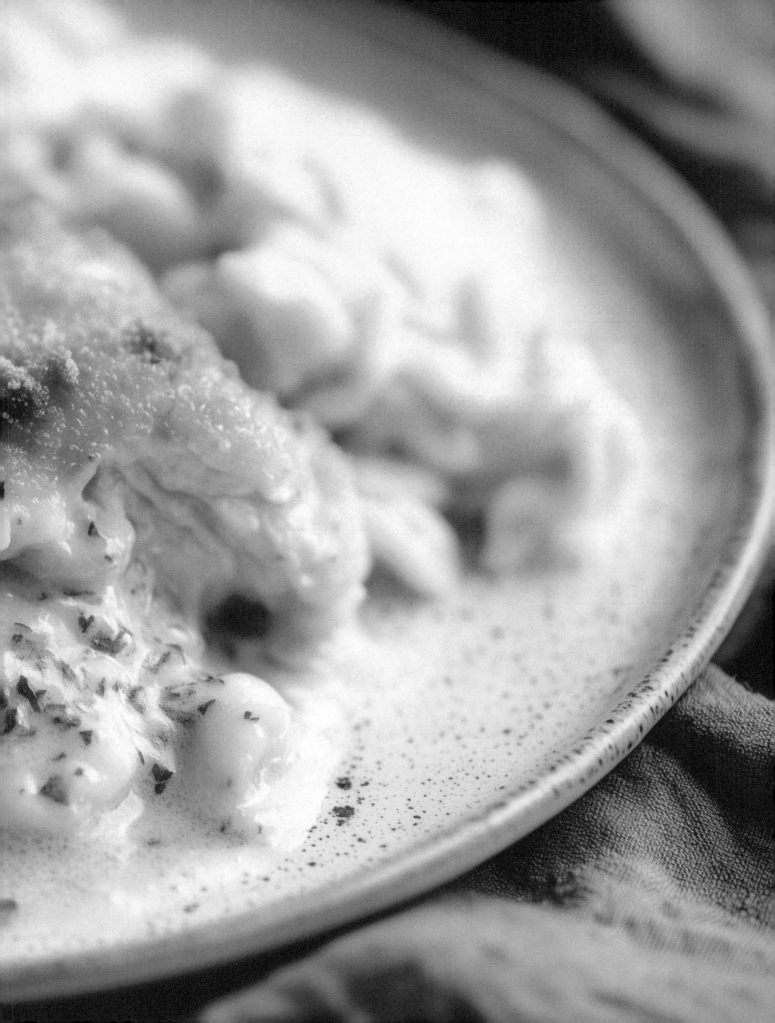

Pork Carnitas Tacos

 Under 30 minutes

INGREDIENTS:

- » ½ cup shredded pork
- » 2 small tortillas
- » 1 tablespoon salsa
- » 1 tablespoon diced onion

INSTRUCTIONS:

1. Warm tortillas in a skillet. Place shredded pork in each tortilla and top with salsa and diced onion.
2. Serve immediately, optionally garnished with fresh cilantro. These pork carnitas tacos are flavorful, tender, and perfect for a quick Mexican-inspired meal with a burst of zest.

NUTRITIONAL VALUES (PER SERVING):

Calories: 300; Protein: 18g; Carbohydrates: 20g; Fiber: 3g; Total Fat: 14g

Spinach and Ricotta Stuffed Shells

 Under 30 minutes

INGREDIENTS:

- » 6 pasta shells, cooked
- » ¼ cup ricotta cheese
- » ¼ cup spinach, chopped
- » 2 tablespoons marinara sauce

INSTRUCTIONS:

1. Preheat oven to 375°F. Mix ricotta and spinach, then fill each pasta shell with the mixture. Place in a baking dish and cover with marinara sauce.
2. Bake for 10-15 minutes until heated through.
3. Serve warm. These spinach and ricotta stuffed shells are creamy, cheesy, and perfect for a quick Italian-inspired dinner.

NUTRITIONAL VALUES (PER SERVING):

Calories: 220; Protein: 10g; Carbohydrates: 25g; Fiber: 2g; Total Fat: 10g

Turkey and Sweet Potato Skillet

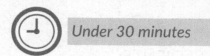 *Under 30 minutes*

INGREDIENTS:

» ½ cup ground turkey
» ½ cup diced sweet potatoes
» 1 tablespoon olive oil
» Salt and pepper to taste

INSTRUCTIONS:

1. In a skillet, heat olive oil over medium heat. Add ground turkey and cook until browned about 5-7 minutes.
2. Add diced sweet potatoes, stirring occasionally until tender, around 10 minutes.
3. Serve warm. This turkey and sweet potato skillet is hearty, flavorful, and perfect for a balanced, nutritious meal.

NUTRITIONAL VALUES (PER SERVING):

Calories: 260; Protein: 18g; Carbohydrates: 20g; Fiber: 3g; Total Fat: 12g

Beef and Cheese Enchiladas

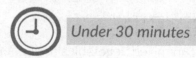 *Under 30 minutes*

INGREDIENTS:

» ½ cup cooked ground beef
» 2 corn tortillas
» ¼ cup shredded cheese
» ¼ cup enchilada sauce

INSTRUCTIONS:

1. Preheat oven to 375°F. Fill each tortilla with beef, roll it up, and place it in a baking dish. Cover with enchilada sauce and sprinkle with cheese.
2. Bake for 15-20 minutes until cheese is melted.
3. Serve hot. These beef and cheese enchiladas are cheesy, flavorful, and perfect for a quick, satisfying meal.

NUTRITIONAL VALUES (PER SERVING):

Calories: 280; Protein: 15g; Carbohydrates: 26g; Fiber: 3g; Total Fat: 14g

Grilled Lamb Chops

 Under 30 minutes

INGREDIENTS:

»   2 lamb chops
»   1 tablespoon olive oil
»   Salt, pepper, and rosemary to taste

INSTRUCTIONS:

1.   Preheat the grill to medium-high heat. Rub lamb chops with olive oil, salt, pepper, and rosemary.
2.   Grill for 4-5 minutes per side until cooked to the desired doneness.
3.   Serve immediately. These grilled lamb chops are tender, flavorful, and perfect for a quick, elegant meal.

NUTRITIONAL VALUES (PER SERVING):

Calories: 320; Protein: 22g; Carbohydrates: 0g; Fiber: 0g; Total Fat: 26g

Vegetarian Thai Red Curry

 Under 30 minutes

INGREDIENTS:

»   ½ cup mixed vegetables (bell peppers, carrots, broccoli)
»   ¼ cup coconut milk
»   1 tablespoon Thai red curry paste

INSTRUCTIONS:

1.   In a pot, combine vegetables, coconut milk, and red curry paste, bringing to a simmer.
2.   Cook for 10-15 minutes until vegetables are tender.
3.   Serve hot over rice. This Thai red curry is creamy, spicy, and perfect for a quick, satisfying vegetarian meal.

NUTRITIONAL VALUES (PER SERVING):

Calories: 180; Protein: 3g; Carbohydrates: 20g; Fiber: 4g; Total Fat: 10g

Spaghetti with Marinara Sauce

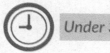 *Under 30 minutes*

INGREDIENTS:

- » 1 cup cooked spaghetti
- » ½ cup marinara sauce
- » Parmesan cheese for garnish

INSTRUCTIONS:

1. In a saucepan, warm the marinara sauce over medium heat.
2. Toss with cooked spaghetti until coated.
3. Serve hot, garnished with Parmesan cheese. This spaghetti with marinara is simple, classic, and perfect for a quick Italian-inspired meal.

NUTRITIONAL VALUES (PER SERVING):

Calories: 280; Protein: 8g; Carbohydrates: 44g; Fiber: 4g; Total Fat: 6g

Chicken Burrito Bowls

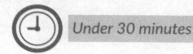 *Under 30 minutes*

INGREDIENTS:

- » ½ cup cooked rice
- » ¼ cup black beans
- » ½ cup cooked chicken, diced
- » 2 tablespoons salsa

INSTRUCTIONS:

1. In a bowl, layer rice, black beans, and chicken.
2. Top with salsa and serve immediately. This chicken burrito bowl is filling, flavorful, and perfect for a quick Mexican-inspired meal that's easy to customize.

NUTRITIONAL VALUES (PER SERVING):

Calories: 300; Protein: 20g; Carbohydrates: 40g; Fiber: 6g; Total Fat: 8g

Shrimp and Grits with Bacon

 Under 30 minutes

INGREDIENTS:

- » ½ cup shrimp, peeled and deveined
- » ¼ cup quick-cooking grits
- » 1 slice bacon, cooked and crumbled
- » 1 tablespoon butter

INSTRUCTIONS:

1. Prepare grits according to package instructions. In a skillet, melt butter and cook shrimp until pink, about 3-4 minutes.
2. Top grits with shrimp and crumbled bacon, stirring to combine.
3. Serve warm. This shrimp and grits with bacon is creamy, savory, and packed with comforting Southern flavors, perfect for a quick yet hearty meal.

NUTRITIONAL VALUES (PER SERVING):

Calories: 280; Protein: 18g; Carbohydrates: 20g; Fiber: 2g; Total Fat: 14g

Chicken Florentine

 Under 30 minutes

INGREDIENTS:

- » 1 chicken breast, sliced
- » 1 cup fresh spinach
- » ¼ cup heavy cream
- » 1 tablespoon olive oil

INSTRUCTIONS:

1. In a skillet, heat olive oil over medium heat and cook chicken until browned.
2. Add spinach and cream, stirring until spinach wilts and sauce thickens.
3. Serve immediately. This chicken Florentine is creamy, rich, and packed with fresh spinach, making it a delicious and easy meal.

NUTRITIONAL VALUES (PER SERVING):

Calories: 320; Protein: 24g; Carbohydrates: 4g; Fiber: 1g; Total Fat: 22g

Baked Mac and Cheese

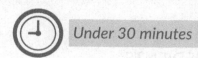 *Under 30 minutes*

INGREDIENTS:

» 1 cup cooked macaroni
» ¼ cup cheddar cheese, shredded
» ¼ cup milk
» 1 tablespoon butter

INSTRUCTIONS:

1. Preheat oven to 375°F. In a baking dish, mix cooked macaroni, milk, butter, and cheddar cheese.
2. Bake for 15-20 minutes until cheese is melted and bubbly.
3. Serve warm. This baked mac and cheese is creamy, cheesy, and comforting, perfect for a quick, hearty meal.

NUTRITIONAL VALUES (PER SERVING):

Calories: 300; Protein: 12g; Carbohydrates: 32g; Fiber: 2g; Total Fat: 16g

Grilled Steak with Chimichurri

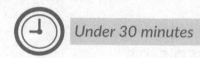 *Under 30 minutes*

INGREDIENTS:

» 1 steak
» 1 tablespoon olive oil
» 1 tablespoon chimichurri sauce

INSTRUCTIONS:

1. Preheat the grill to medium-high heat. Brush steak with olive oil and grill for 4-5 minutes per side until desired doneness.
2. Let rest briefly, then slice and top with chimichurri sauce.
3. Serve hot. This grilled steak with chimichurri is juicy, flavorful, and perfect for a quick, satisfying meal with a tangy twist.

NUTRITIONAL VALUES (PER SERVING):

Calories: 340; Protein: 24g; Carbohydrates: 2g; Fiber: 0g; Total Fat: 26g

Stuffed Mushrooms

 Under 30 minutes

INGREDIENTS:

- »   6 large mushrooms, stems removed
- »   ¼ cup cream cheese
- »   1 tablespoon Parmesan cheese
- »   1 clove garlic, minced

INSTRUCTIONS:

1. Preheat oven to 375°F. In a bowl, mix cream cheese, Parmesan, and garlic, then spoon into mushroom caps.
2. Bake for 15-20 minutes until mushrooms are tender.
3. Serve warm. These stuffed mushrooms are creamy, garlicky, and perfect as a quick appetizer or light meal.

NUTRITIONAL VALUES (PER SERVING):

Calories: 120; Protein: 4g; Carbohydrates: 6g; Fiber: 2g; Total Fat: 10g

Vegan Lentil Soup

 Under 30 minutes

INGREDIENTS:

- »   ½ cup lentils
- »   1 cup vegetable broth
- »   ¼ cup diced carrots
- »   ¼ cup diced celery

INSTRUCTIONS:

1. In a pot, combine lentils, vegetable broth, carrots, and celery. Bring to a boil, then simmer for 20 minutes until lentils are tender.
2. Serve warm, optionally garnished with fresh herbs. This vegan lentil soup is hearty, nutritious, and perfect for a quick plant-based meal.

NUTRITIONAL VALUES (PER SERVING):

Calories: 180; Protein: 10g; Carbohydrates: 28g; Fiber: 8g; Total Fat: 2g

Baked Zucchini with Cheese

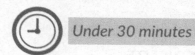 *Under 30 minutes*

INGREDIENTS:

- » 1 zucchini, sliced
- » ¼ cup shredded mozzarella
- » 1 tablespoon Parmesan cheese
- » Salt and pepper to taste

INSTRUCTIONS:

1. Preheat oven to 400°F. Arrange zucchini slices on a baking sheet, season with salt and pepper, and sprinkle with mozzarella and Parmesan.
2. Bake for 12-15 minutes until cheese is melted and golden.
3. Serve warm. This baked zucchini with cheese is light, savory, and a perfect quick side dish.

NUTRITIONAL VALUES (PER SERVING):

Calories: 100; Protein: 6g; Carbohydrates: 4g; Fiber: 1g; Total Fat: 7g

Chicken and Pesto Flatbread

 Under 30 minutes

INGREDIENTS:

- » 1 small flatbread
- » ¼ cup cooked chicken, shredded
- » 2 tablespoons pesto sauce
- » ¼ cup mozzarella cheese, shredded

INSTRUCTIONS:

1. Preheat oven to 400°F. Spread pesto sauce on the flatbread, then top with chicken and mozzarella.
2. Bake for 10-12 minutes until cheese is melted and bubbly.
3. Serve warm. This chicken and pesto flatbread is flavorful, cheesy, and ideal for a quick meal with Italian flair.

NUTRITIONAL VALUES (PER SERVING):

Calories: 250; Protein: 14g; Carbohydrates: 24g; Fiber: 1g; Total Fat: 10g

Pesto Tortellini

 Under 30 minutes

INGREDIENTS:

- » 1 cup cheese tortellini, cooked
- » 2 tablespoons pesto sauce
- » Parmesan cheese for garnish

INSTRUCTIONS:

1. In a large bowl, toss cooked tortellini with pesto sauce until evenly coated.
2. Serve warm, garnished with Parmesan cheese if desired.
3. This pesto tortellini is creamy, fresh, and a quick Italian-inspired meal that's easy and satisfying.

NUTRITIONAL VALUES (PER SERVING):

Calories: 320; Protein: 12g; Carbohydrates: 34g; Fiber: 2g; Total Fat: 14g

Lamb Stew

 Under 30 minutes

INGREDIENTS:

- » ½ cup diced lamb
- » ½ cup diced carrots and potatoes
- » 1 cup beef broth

INSTRUCTIONS:

1. In a pot, combine lamb, carrots, potatoes, and beef broth. Bring to a boil, then simmer for 20 minutes until the lamb is tender and flavors are blended.
2. Serve hot. This lamb stew is hearty, savory, and perfect for a quick, comforting meal with rich flavors.

NUTRITIONAL VALUES (PER SERVING):

Calories: 300; Protein: 20g; Carbohydrates: 20g; Fiber: 3g; Total Fat: 14g

Roasted Beet Salad

 Under 30 minutes

INGREDIENTS:

» 1 cup roasted beets, diced
» ¼ cup feta cheese, crumbled
» 1 tablespoon balsamic vinegar
» 1 tablespoon olive oil

INSTRUCTIONS:

1. Arrange roasted beets on a plate and sprinkle with crumbled feta.
2. Drizzle with balsamic vinegar and olive oil, then toss gently to combine.
3. Serve immediately. This roasted beet salad is earthy, tangy, and perfect as a refreshing, colorful dish full of vibrant flavors and textures.

NUTRITIONAL VALUES (PER SERVING):

Calories: 180; Protein: 5g; Carbohydrates: 16g; Fiber: 4g; Total Fat: 10g

Beef Tacos with Salsa

 Under 30 minutes

INGREDIENTS:

» ½ cup cooked ground beef
» 2 small tortillas
» 2 tablespoons salsa
» 1 tablespoon diced onion

INSTRUCTIONS:

1. Place cooked ground beef on each tortilla. Top with salsa and diced onion.
2. Serve immediately, optionally garnished with cilantro or cheese. These beef tacos with salsa are flavorful, easy to prepare, and perfect for a quick, satisfying meal with a bit of spice.

NUTRITIONAL VALUES (PER SERVING):

Calories: 300; Protein: 15g; Carbohydrates: 24g; Fiber: 2g; Total Fat: 16g

Roasted Chicken with Thyme

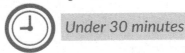 *Under 30 minutes*

INGREDIENTS:

» 1 chicken thigh
» 1 tablespoon olive oil
» 1 teaspoon fresh thyme leaves
» Salt and pepper to taste

INSTRUCTIONS:

1. Preheat oven to 400°F. Rub chicken with olive oil, thyme, salt, and pepper.
2. Roast in the oven for 20-25 minutes until cooked through and golden.
3. Serve hot. This roasted chicken with thyme is aromatic, tender, and perfect for a quick, hearty meal with a touch of herbaceous flavor.

NUTRITIONAL VALUES (PER SERVING):

Calories: 220; Protein: 20g; Carbohydrates: 0g; Fiber: 0g; Total Fat: 14g

Soba Noodles with Veggies

 Under 30 minutes

INGREDIENTS:

» 1 cup cooked soba noodles
» ½ cup mixed vegetables (bell peppers, carrots, snap peas)
» 1 tablespoon soy sauce
» 1 teaspoon sesame oil

INSTRUCTIONS:

1. In a skillet, heat sesame oil over medium heat and add mixed vegetables, cooking until tender-crisp.
2. Toss with soba noodles and soy sauce until evenly combined.
3. Serve warm. This soba noodle dish is light, flavorful, and full of nutritious vegetables, ideal for a quick, satisfying meal.

NUTRITIONAL VALUES (PER SERVING):

Calories: 250; Protein: 8g; Carbohydrates: 40g; Fiber: 4g; Total Fat: 8g

Grilled Salmon with Mango Salsa

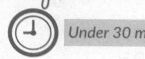 *Under 30 minutes*

INGREDIENTS:

» 1 salmon fillet
» ¼ cup diced mango
» 1 tablespoon diced red onion
» 1 tablespoon lime juice

INSTRUCTIONS:

1. Grill salmon over medium heat for 10-12 minutes until cooked through.
2. In a small bowl, mix mango, red onion, and lime juice. Spoon salsa over grilled salmon before serving.
3. This grilled salmon with mango salsa is fresh, tangy, and perfect for a quick, flavorful dinner.

NUTRITIONAL VALUES (PER SERVING):

Calories: 280; Protein: 22g; Carbohydrates: 12g; Fiber: 2g; Total Fat: 16g

Pork and Apple Skewers

 Under 30 minutes

INGREDIENTS:

» ½ cup pork tenderloin, cubed
» ½ apple, cubed
» 1 tablespoon olive oil
» Salt and pepper to taste

INSTRUCTIONS:

1. Thread pork and apple cubes onto skewers, brush with olive oil, and season with salt and pepper.
2. Grill over medium heat for 8-10 minutes, turning occasionally until pork is cooked through.
3. Serve immediately. These pork and apple skewers are savory and slightly sweet, making for a perfect quick meal or appetizer.

NUTRITIONAL VALUES (PER SERVING):

Calories: 200; Protein: 15g; Carbohydrates: 8g; Fiber: 1g; Total Fat: 10g

Shrimp Tacos with Avocado Salsa

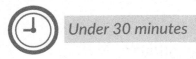
Under 30 minutes

INGREDIENTS:

» ½ cup shrimp, cooked and peeled
» 2 small tortillas
» ¼ avocado, diced
» 1 tablespoon diced tomato

INSTRUCTIONS:

1. Place shrimp on each tortilla. In a small bowl, mix diced avocado and tomato to create salsa.
2. Spoon salsa over the shrimp and serve immediately. These shrimp tacos with avocado salsa are fresh, light, and perfect for a quick, tropical-inspired meal.

NUTRITIONAL VALUES (PER SERVING):

Calories: 230; Protein: 14g; Carbohydrates: 20g; Fiber: 3g; Total Fat: 10g

Baked Eggplant Parmesan

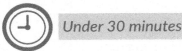
Under 30 minutes

INGREDIENTS:

» 1 small eggplant, sliced
» ¼ cup marinara sauce
» ¼ cup shredded mozzarella
» 1 tablespoon Parmesan cheese

INSTRUCTIONS:

1. Preheat oven to 375°F. Place eggplant slices on a baking sheet and top with marinara and cheese.
2. Bake for 15-20 minutes until cheese is bubbly and golden.
3. Serve hot. This baked eggplant Parmesan is cheesy, hearty, and ideal for a quick Italian-inspired meal.

NUTRITIONAL VALUES (PER SERVING):

Calories: 200; Protein: 8g; Carbohydrates: 16g; Fiber: 5g; Total Fat: 12g

Vegetarian Lasagna

 Under 30 minutes

INGREDIENTS:

- » 2 lasagna noodles, cooked
- » ¼ cup ricotta cheese
- » ¼ cup spinach, chopped
- » ¼ cup marinara sauce

INSTRUCTIONS:

1. Preheat oven to 375°F. Layer lasagna noodles with ricotta, spinach, and marinara in a small baking dish.
2. Bake for 15-20 minutes until heated through.
3. Serve hot. This vegetarian lasagna is creamy, cheesy, and perfect for a quick, satisfying, meatless dinner.

NUTRITIONAL VALUES (PER SERVING):

Calories: 240; Protein: 10g; Carbohydrates: 30g; Fiber: 4g; Total Fat: 8g

Bbq Pulled Pork

 Under 30 minutes

INGREDIENTS:

- » ½ cup shredded cooked pork
- » 2 tablespoons BBQ sauce
- » 1 sandwich roll

INSTRUCTIONS:

1. In a skillet, heat shredded pork with BBQ sauce until warm and evenly coated.
2. Serve on a sandwich roll, optionally topped with coleslaw.
3. This BBQ pulled pork is smoky, tangy, and perfect for a quick, satisfying meal with classic barbecue flavors.

NUTRITIONAL VALUES (PER SERVING):

Calories: 300; Protein: 15g; Carbohydrates: 34g; Fiber: 2g; Total Fat: 12g

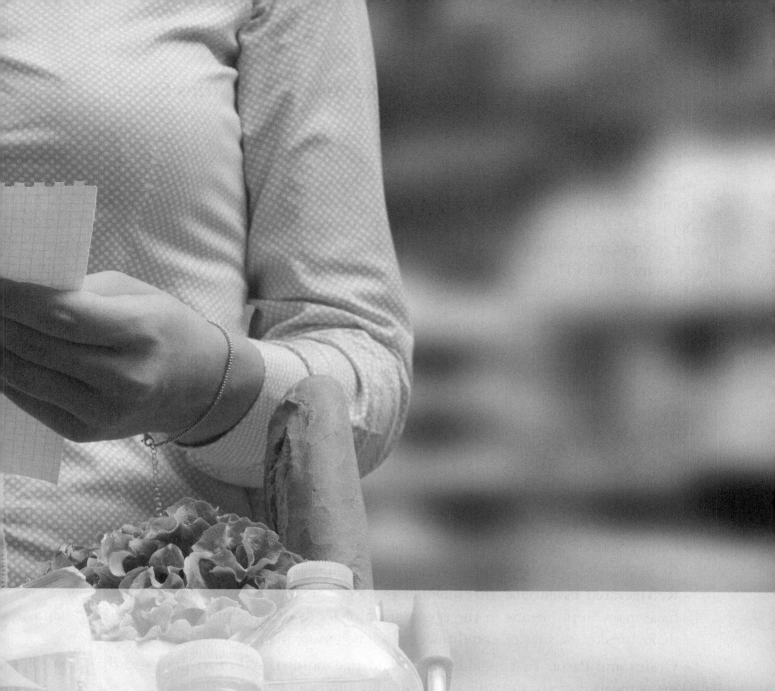

Bonus Section

Downloadable Shopping List

PDF Shopping List to Make Your Grocery Trips Easier

An organized shopping list is very helpful when it comes to food preparation, and this book contains all that is needed in order to make shopping an interesting affair. For every recipe, you'll see a clear list of what you will need to make it, so there is no confusion as to what you have to buy. To make it even easier for you, we have developed a PDF shopping list that lists the basic pantry items that you should always have on hand so that if you want to cook something mouth-watering, you are always ready for the task. With a clear list for each recipe and a PDF, you can either save or print. You should be ready to go grocery shopping, which should help to take the stress out of proper meal preparation.

The PDF is actually a neatly compiled list of pantry items, fresh produce, and household items used day to day, which will greatly assist those with tight schedules. This category encompasses food that contains long life, such as olive oil, spices, fresh herbs, and grains, as well as proteins like chicken and tofu, among others. Most of these are semi-perishable and used in many recipes, so always ensuring you have stock will save you time in the food store while you relax in the kitchen preparing the meals.

How to Use Your PDF Shopping List

The downloadable PDF is rightly categorized, and therefore, there is hardly any fuss in finding any of the items. Below are some of the sections you'll find in the list:

- **Pantry Staples:** Simple staples such as olive oil, vinegar, salt, pepper, and regular spices. With these on hand, you can easily cook different recipes ranging from sauces to spice mixtures.

- **Refrigerated Essentials:** This includes products such as milk, butter, eggs, and yogurt that have many applications in the preparation of foods. It is helpful to have these on hand to make breakfasts, snacks, and dinner prep much more manageable.

- **Grains and Pasta:** That includes pasta and rice, quinoa, and other grains so that a base for many meals is ready and no last-minute shopping will be needed.

- **Proteins:** It is important to have a choice of different proteins, and for that, it is necessary to have chicken breasts and ground beef as well as tofu and chickpeas for various meals throughout the week.

- **Produce:** A long list of fresh vegetables and fruits often used in recipes, starting with onions and bell peppers and moving to garlic, spinach, and arugula. Thus, all you need for salads, stir-fries, and garnishing would be nearby, where you handle most of your food preparation.

- **Dairy and Non-Dairy Options:** Cheese, milk, and yogurt are included, along with non-dairy alternatives like almond or oat milk for those who prefer or need dairy-free options.

Customizing Your Shopping List

The bottom of the PDF also includes a section called notes, in which you can specify amounts based on servings in case you need smaller portions. I find this to be a great feature, especially when preparing for a household of one, a family, or even when feeding a number of friends.

Benefits of Using the PDF Shopping List:

- **Efficiency:** It means forgetting certain essences or walking around the store aimlessly searching for something to put inside the kitchen. The list helps you stay focused, especially if you are operating on a budget.
- **Consistency:** Ensuring you have the basics stocked allows you to confidently approach each recipe without last-minute substitutions or omissions.
- **Reduced Waste:** When you know exactly what you'll use in the week, it's easier to buy only what you need, minimizing food waste and making the most of each grocery trip.

Having a clear shopping list with all the ingredients required for the recipes in this book saves you time and reduces the stress of meal planning. It can be daunting to think of all the items needed to cook a variety of meals in a week, but with this PDF, you'll feel prepared and organized.

Using the List to Prep for Different Meals

How can the meals be prepped? Well, with this kind of sequence in place, you'll find that meal prepping is a completely stress-free process. For instance, whenever you are designing a weekly meal plan for the purpose of cooking, start by going through all the recipes featured in this book and matching them to the ingredients listed on the PDF shopping list devised above. In this way, you have all that you may need during the day, this or the other thing, and you don't need to go out repeatedly; after that, you risk forgetting something significant.

What is more, if you wanted to make things even easier, you could also group meals of the week around some of those basics. For instance, a single purchase of pasta could be divided into multiple meals, such as Pasta with Marinara Sauce on one night, Pasta Primavera on another, and Pesto Tortellini later in the week. Similarly, purchasing a bag of spinach could serve as the base for Spinach Lasagna Rolls, an addition to a Chicken Florentine, and a salad mix-in.

Staple Ingredients to Keep on Hand

The PDF includes a list of items that are commonly used across recipes and are good to have on hand at all times. Stocking your pantry with these basics will help you adapt to different recipes and minimize unexpected trips to the store. Here are some examples of staple ingredients:

1. **Spices and Seasonings:** Salt, pepper, garlic powder, onion powder, Italian seasoning, cumin, paprika, and chili powder are included as they form the foundation of many dishes.
2. **Herbs:** Fresh herbs like basil, cilantro, and parsley are essential for adding flavor and freshness to your dishes.

3. **Oils and Vinegar:** Olive oil, vegetable oil, balsamic vinegar, and apple cider vinegar allow you to prepare dressings, marinades, and sautéed dishes easily.

4. **Baking Essentials:** Items like flour, baking powder, and baking soda are useful not only for baked goods but also for thickening sauces and adding texture to dishes.

5. **Canned Goods:** Tomato paste, diced tomatoes, black beans, and chickpeas provide a versatile base for various recipes, from soups to chili to salads.

Weekly Grocery Planning Tips

1. **Plan Recipes Ahead:** Browse the recipes in this book and select your weekly meals in advance. Use the shopping list to identify what you already have at home and what you need to purchase.

2. **Check for Seasonal Produce:** Indeed, some of the items on this list are general, but changing due to the seasons of fruits and vegetables makes it routine and fresh. One should be more creative in the choice of dishes, aiming at using products that are cheaper when in season in salads, soups, and side dishes.

3. **Choose Multi-Use Ingredients:** Products that are reusable in different recipes make your shopping expeditions more productive and less costly. Such things as bell peppers can be consumed in stir-fries, salads, or fajitas.

Printable and Digital PDF for Convenience

The PDF shopping list is in A4 format, which again has an option to print the list or view it on a phone/tablet device. An option digitized is particularly useful if you will otherwise cross off items as you shop or change quantities based on specific meals.

In this sense, shopping in this manner of selecting meals and grouping foods helps to optimize the use of ingredients, reduce waste, and make cooking easier. Really, it's all about making your lives easier by helping build time around a specific meal type and not having to stop at the grocery store at the last second. The PDF Shopping List has been created to be a handy sidekick that helps you plan and make lists and keeps you motivated to cook.

With every recipe, a cooking list, and a printable PDF of all the common items needed for your meals, meal planning is a fun and simple event. The PDF is not only a recipe book but also a reference to encourage a daily/weekly/monthly systematic manner about buying food and practicing cooking. So this neatly divided and categorized list is perfect whether you are setting up a week's grocery shopping, introducing a new dish into the household, or just topping up the provisions. The convenience of having all the needed ingredients for any and every single recipe you would attempt in this book and another great factor is that you know it's safe for consumption.

Budget-Friendly Guide to Keeping Your Pantry Stocked

Cheap, useful ingredients are the main keyword of this book, as they are going to allow the author to save on groceries while using the ingredients for as many dishes as possible. This should be done while denying yourself the luxuries of exotic or single-serving items that end up contributing to your grocery bill yet are rarely used once they get home. On the contrary, the recipes given here use ingredients that are easily found and can add a lot of change and diversification to your meals without asking for all sorts of spices and condiments.

Stocking your pantry is one of the ways of reducing costs regarding meal preparation. Products such as pasta, rice, beans, canned tomatoes, and regular-use spices are cheap to obtain, easy to stock, and flexible to use given various dishes. Buying these necessity items whenever they are out of offer or cheaper than usual means of saving is all other than rational as it also means saving on the number of visits that are made to the grocery stores. This book also illustrates how these staple pantry ingredients can be combined again and again to prepare tasty and healthy meals.

Each time you are purchasing raw materials for your pantry, it is wise to go for products with extended shelf life. Basic ingredients like olive oil, dried herbs, pasta, and grains can be used for months, allowing you to cook a meal anytime you want. As for frozen products, we should also note that they are more economical since they take little time to freeze and are as versatile as fresh fruits and vegetables. However, canned foods such as beans and diced tomatoes are pretty versatile in the kitchen and easily storable for quick and cheap meal preparation.

This approach to stocking a pantry can also help reduce food waste. When your ingredients can be used in multiple dishes, there's less risk of them going to waste. For example, a bag of rice can serve as a base for stir-fries, burrito bowls, and side dishes, while pasta can be dressed up with different sauces, vegetables, and proteins for an entirely new flavor profile each time. By buying versatile ingredients, you also simplify the decision-making process. When your pantry is filled with multi-use items, creating a meal becomes more about combining flavors than following a rigid recipe.

Using what you already have on hand and making slight adjustments to recipes is a great way to stretch your budget further. For instance, if a recipe calls for bell peppers and you have carrots instead, feel free to make that substitution. Many vegetables are interchangeable in recipes like stir-fries, soups, and salads, so you don't need to buy every item listed if a similar option is available. This flexibility not only saves money but also reduces stress, allowing you to focus on enjoying the cooking process rather than worrying about having every exact ingredient.

Another advantage of stocking your pantry with such ingredients is that this way, you start learning to be creative in the kitchen. When you realize that all recipes except a few are flexible enough and can be used interchangeably, the creativity floor is opened. Occasionally, you realize that getting grains such as quinoa and combining them with canned beans plus fresh vegetables will make you a healthy meal that you cannot buy elsewhere. Just as tomato sauce or pesto can turn pasta, rice, or roasted vegetables into quite a tasty dish with relative ease, it is trying to understand how to come up with new combinations of these basics so as to ensure that you do not spend a lot of time and a lot of money preparing different meals.

Maintaining a budget for many people is about saying no to additional expenses on any luxury or special products, and this can be demotivating. But, what is interesting is that whilst you're rationed with what's inside your pantry, you will realize that there is a great deal of versatility. Meat tenderizers and herbs and spices are cheap items that make a big difference in your cooking by adding heat to your pots. Even a teaspoon of garlic powder, paprika, cumin, and oregano go a long way in altering the taste of your dish, whether it's you are roasting vegetables or preparing soup. It only takes a small prop, and those are easy to purchase and incorporate into meals at minimal cost.

They mean that when you set your week's meal, you have to accommodate the products that you already have, hence using them efficiently. For instance, when you prefer a jar of marinara sauce, know that they are not only for pasta meal preparation. Marinara can be used to prepare a pizza sauce, add a topping to baked chicken, or simply serve as a dipping sauce for breadsticks. Likewise, besides being used in baking, a bag of flour contains many other uses, including breading meat before frying, as a thickener for sauces, or as the base for homemade tortillas or flatbreads.

One of the best ways to get into the habit of using pantry staples effectively is to set a weekly menu based on what you have on hand. If you notice that you have a lot of rice, plan for meals that incorporate it as a side dish or main component, like rice bowls, fried rice, or stuffed bell peppers. Over time, you'll develop a sense of what ingredients work well together and what items are worth keeping stocked so your pantry becomes a resource rather than just storage.

Maintaining the costs might mean the difference between cutting down on expensive proteins or buying cheap vegetables in a certain period. Eggs, beans, and canned tuna are other good and cheap sources of protein that you can use in almost any dish. For instance, beans are very flexible and can be incorporated in tacos, stews, and salads, as well as a grainier alternative. By deciding on such sorts of ingredients, you have an opportunity to please your stomach while not having a feeling that everything is limited.

Also, the purchasing of materials in large quantities is advisable for essentials and other products, which are often used for a long time. Rice, pasta, and dried pulses are good examples of foods that one usually buys in large quantities, and putting them in can easily whip up a meal at short notice. When you are preparing your meals, you will always have a base from which to start, depending on whether you fancy stir-fried pasta or soup.

You also find yourself going out to buy more ingredients more frequently when your pantry is not well-stocked, especially with cheap ingredients. So, should you ever find yourself in a bit of a culinary crisis, you will only need to check your pantry and freezer to create a wholesome, satisfying meal without breaking the bank. What can be found at home, like frozen vegetables, canned vegetables, and pasta, provide you with a means of preparing pasta primavera or vegetable soups without having to use fresh produce. These options are flexible and minimize wastage because frozen and canned products last for many months.

Cooking on a budget doesn't mean you have to sacrifice quality or flavor. In fact, many simple ingredients, like garlic, onions, and fresh herbs, provide a lot of taste without a high cost. By using these flavor enhancers in different recipes, you can create diverse and satisfying meals that don't require expensive or hard-to-find ingredients. A pinch of red pepper flakes, a squeeze of lemon juice, or a dash of soy sauce can transform a dish, adding brightness, heat, or umami without the need for specialty items.

Moreover, if you buy oils and vinegar and other grains that you want to cook for the family, you make yourself ready to cook for the family. An excellent olive oil, as an illustration, can be employed in sautéing foods, dressing on salad, or incorporating it into sauces. Likewise, balsamic vinegar or apple cider vinegar is also appropriate in marinades, dressings, and glazes. They not only bring the flavor but also help you produce something out of the other things you have bought, thus maximizing your grocery expenses.

Another way to maximize your budget is by prepping and freezing items when you have an abundance. If you find fresh vegetables on sale, consider chopping and freezing them for later use in soups, stir-fries, or casseroles. This way, you're not wasting produce, and you have a supply ready for future meals. Herbs can also be frozen in olive oil or butter for easy use in cooking, preserving their flavor and reducing waste.

Last of all, having a pantry filled with store-bought basic ingredients that are inexpensive puts a hold on stressing over what to have for a meal. If your pantry is stocked with a variety of staple foods that are used in most recipes, you will always be able to choose to cook different meals using the ingredients on hand and experiment with recipes. That way, you are able to grow more independent and relaxed about preparing the meals within your means instead of being limited to a price range.

Focusing on some staple foods and ingredients, this book is designed to help make cooking fun, easy, and financially painless. Fuss over preparing large meals daily, with a few wisely selected items; you can make meals that correspond to different tastes and preferences as well as to calories consumed. Adopting such a strategy actually pays off, but more importantly, it encourages people to cook mindfully, avoiding wastage in the whole process. Whether you're a professional chef or a student who cooks pumpkin, this guide to a budget pantry is here to help create delicious meals without using many dollars.

SCAN THIS QR CODE TO ACCESS YOUR BONUSES!

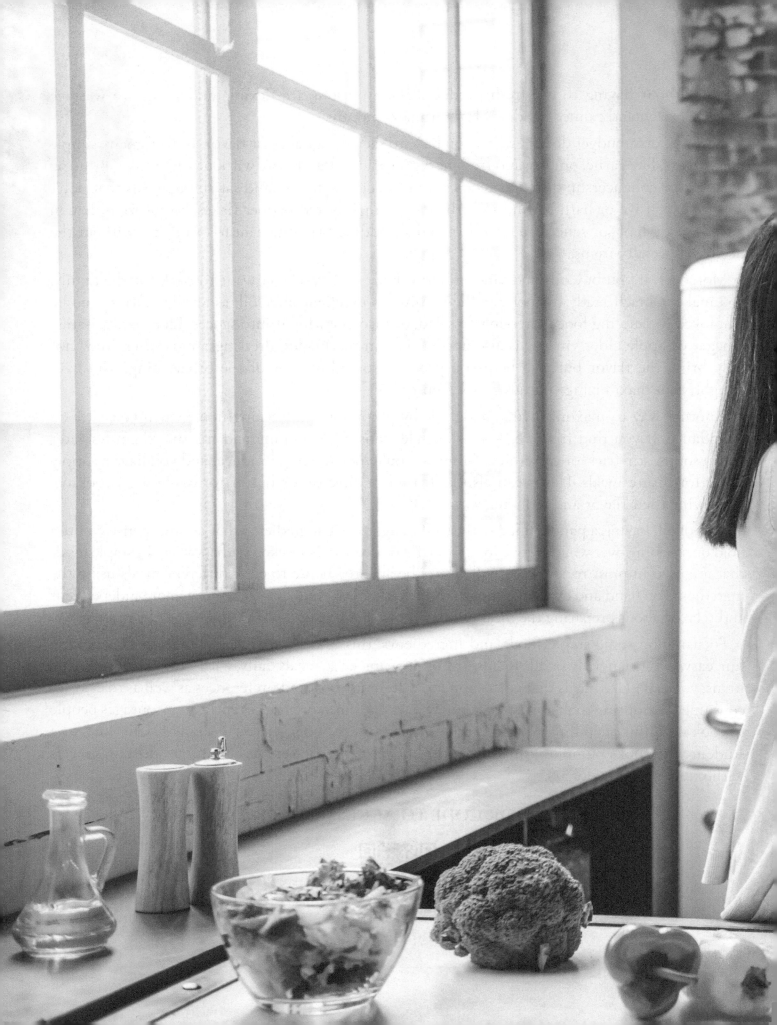

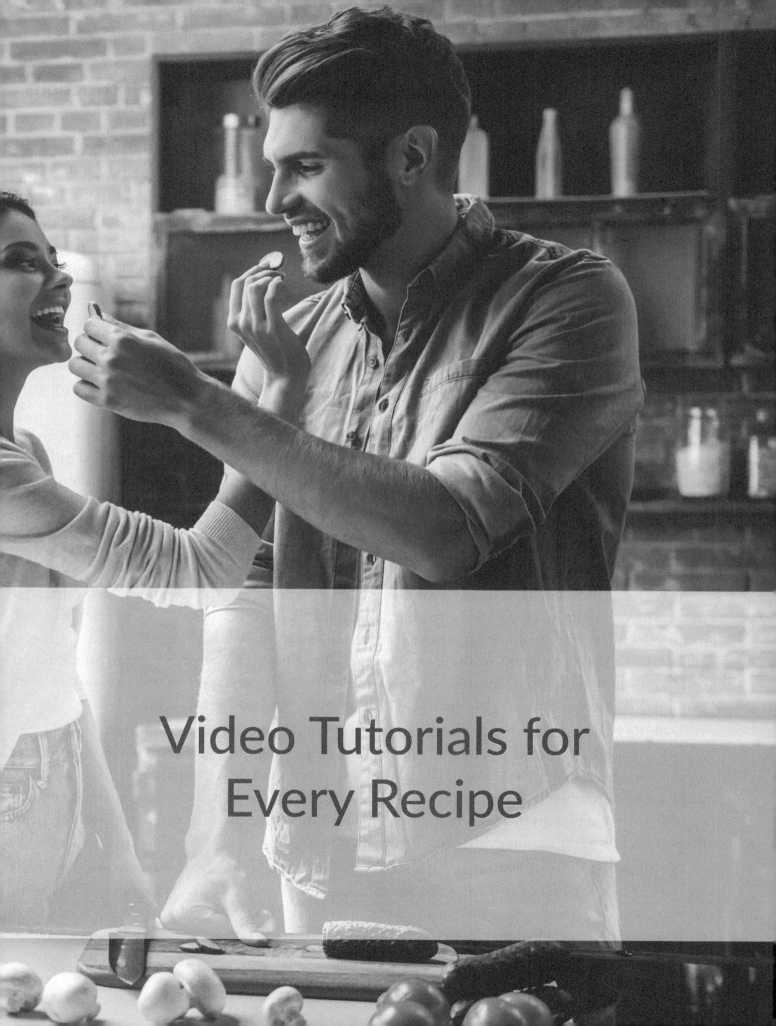

Video Tutorials for
Every Recipe

Learn How to Cook Each Recipe with Quick and Easy Video Instructions

In addition to clear written instructions, each recipe in this book has a video demonstration intended to help the reader through every stage. In any of the recipes, experienced cooks, as well as novices, can easily follow along and cook the meals to perfection. At some point, cooking appears to be very daunting, particularly when preparing a new meal, but having the video makes it less daunting because it guides one in the right manner. Indeed, from how to chop vegetables to what it takes to brown a piece of beef properly, each and every video tutorial is deliberately designed to break down the most intricate process so that a viewer can easily follow an outlined recipe.

These tutorials are for a basic level, and each step is made simple in order to make understanding them easier. We know that everyone learns differently, and while the recipe below is perfect, watching it happen before your very eyes can help you with even the most difficult steps. Each video is split into convenient portions that allow you to cook without progressing through a recipe too quickly, thus losing any details of the process.

Every single one of them is strictly under 10 minutes, so that it covers just enough steps to make you go from the beginning to the very end without including extra information. All significant changes are made to align us with your expectations, which makes the whole process less confusing without adding unnecessary steps. These are basic cooking lessons: from learning about kneading the dough to cooking your own bread to learning how to get a creamy texture for pasta or how to combine flavors in a stew, these videos are created with the purpose of providing the help you need without making the situation look more complicated than it has to be.

As for most individuals, cooking is more of a discovery and trial. The techniques demonstrated in the videos might make you want to change or tweak the recipes to your own preference. For instance, while a tutorial showing how to fry vegetables can show you the general technique, you may feel prompted to bring in some of the vegetables or spices you prefer from your kitchen instead of those demonstrated. It's our passion to help you become an empowered cook in your own kitchen, providing you with the tools to create each meal your own.

Cooking is also a sensory experience, and the videos help you visualize important details that are sometimes hard to convey in text, such as how a sauce should look when it's thickened, the ideal color of caramelized onions, or the proper texture of a finished dish. These small details can make a big difference in the final result, and having a visual reference means you can feel more confident that you're on the right track. Even for beginners, the tutorials offer the assurance that they can achieve restaurant-quality results by following along.

In addition to the videos, there are also some recommendations on how to prepare each ingredient and save time. If during the preparation of dishes, use instructions or some tips on how to chop save time, these are mentioned in the tutorial. This helps you not only get acquainted with how to prepare certain recipes but also acquire features that you can use in different recipes.

For instance, a tutorial on fast and safe slicing of onions enables one to prepare it in many recipes and enhance the cooking experience.

Besides that, the lessons are divided according to the level of complexity, meaning it will be quite easy for you to find something you have never tried before but are still within your technical abilities if any meals or dishes seem to be too difficult for you. Composed recipes, which can be complicated when getting to the actual cooking process, are given simpler steps to make you do not get embarrassed. These videos are a great convenience, especially for newcomers to the culinary world, as they make you sure of what you generally would not attempt to cook.

For those who are experienced, the videos can come in handy as references or even powerful motivators to incorporate personal style. Despite the fact that people who cook often revisit the same recipes, even experienced participants may require some reference information to refresh their memory about certain procedures they engage in or get a new perspective on certain dishes that have already been prepared at one point. The tutorials are helpful in the sense that they give just enough instruction so the drawings are not confusing but enough leeway so that one is still able to create whatever they want.

All the tunes are concept-based, showing the whole process of preparing a dish from start to finish and easy decoration ideas for your creations. Here, you will also learn little details, such as sprinkling fresh herbs on the dish, drawing with a sauce, or placing ingredients on the dish, thinking about their aesthetic appeal. Often, these little tweaks can certainly enrich a dish; sometimes, the presentation can make the process of serving food more engaging and fun, whether cooking for yourself, your loved ones, or even guests.

The other advantage of the video format is that it is flexible. Since it is a streaming-based application, you can watch it on your tablet, which is placed in the kitchen, or the phone put on a stand or, if you like, a large-screen TV. The tutorials are easy to follow, anytime and anyplace, so they enable you to adapt the process of cooking to your own convenience.

There is also guidance for those who may have issues with certain ingredients, and such videos feature demonstrations on how to substitute these ingredients, which are, of course, conceivable. They also show you how to incorporate changes such as going gluten-free, using plants as substitutes, or making low-calorie foods while still having them turn out well. For instance, if the recipe has dairy, then the video might recommend either coconut milk or almond milk in case one wants a low-cream or non-dairy recipe, respectively.

Meal preparation and cooking are not solitary exercises most of the time, and these video tutorials can help make cooking a fun pastime for family or friends. You could watch the videos in pairs or as a group, divide the tasks among the listeners, or cook different dishes with the help of the recipes. It is a good opportunity to make cooking not such an individual job and something people do in their free time that can actually be fun. For parents, the videos can also be informative, extend an invitation to the kids to get involved in the process of preparing meals and educate them on the importance of homemade food.

In addition to the tutorials on the process of cooking, there are also cleaning tips to make the kitchen clean. Every video focuses on how to clean up well, right from reordering bowls and utensils during cooking to reducing clutter as you cook. By implementing these tips, we want to make every step, from the cutting board to the stovetop to the dinner table to the dishwasher, as enjoyable and as easy as we can.

It turned out that each video tutorial is a compiled lesson where the given one mainly contained not only the pure recipe but also the information about the ingredients used in the dish, some techniques used during the show, as well as some useful tips that do not necessarily relate directly to the given dish. Not only will you know how to make each meal by watching the videos, but you also expand the so-called 'emerging kitchen skills,' which contribute to your general performance as a cook. In creating these tutorials, it is assumed that preparing food should be a rewarding process, and you are not alone.

The tutorials are equally useful in today's world, particularly given that they are brief. We understand that some people who came to seek help from us would only spare a few minutes to have a look at these instructions, which is why we do not make the videos long-winded and put all the necessary information in them as briefly and explicitly as possible. It's time effective, meaning one can hustle to prepare a homecooked meal without having to spend much of their day cooking.

Video tutorials enhance this cookbook and turn it into an improved cooking companion with extra help in the form of moving pictures. It's not recipes you're reading; it's recipes in action, which makes the cooking experience logical, fun, and healthy. They are here to make you a better cook, to spark your imagination, and to guarantee that your food will always look and taste as good as the food in these pictures.

SCAN THIS QR CODE TO ACCESS YOUR BONUSES!

Unit Conversion

The unit conversion page included in this book is designed to make following recipes easier, no matter which measurement system you're accustomed to. Cooking measurements can vary significantly, especially between metric and US systems, and this can sometimes create confusion. For example, a recipe might call for ounces or pounds, but you may prefer to measure in grams or vice versa. This page provides easy conversions for weight, volume, temperature, and even length, helping you tackle any recipe with confidence.

Weight Conversions

For dry ingredients like flour, sugar, or spices, weight is usually measured in ounces or pounds in the US and in grams or kilograms in the metric system. Below are some common conversions to help bridge these two systems:

- **1 ounce (oz)** = 28 grams (g)
- **1 pound (lb)** = 454 grams (g)
- **1 cup of flour** = approximately 125 grams (g)
- **1 cup of sugar** = approximately 200 grams (g)

These conversions come in handy more often, especially when baking, where measurements are critically important. For example, flour expressed in grams instead of cups allows for a perfect consistency of the dough for your pastries.

Volume Conversions

For liquids, such measurements include cups, tablespoons, and teaspoons in US Standard practices, as well as milliliters or liters for the metric system. Here are some of the most common conversions to simplify your measurements:

- **1 cup** = 8 fluid ounces (fl oz) = 237 milliliters (ml)
- **1 tablespoon (tbsp)** = 15 milliliters (ml)
- **1 teaspoon (tsp)** = 5 milliliters (ml)

Some of these conversions are useful for almost all types of recipes, from gravies and sauces to soups. When measuring large amounts such as broth or water, it is far easier and more accurate if you have a jug that contains metric measurements in Litres.

Temperature Conversions

This is something about heat treatment, especially in cooking and baking, and ovens use a scale of either Fahrenheit or Celsius. Here's a quick guide for converting between the two:

- **300°F** = 150°C
- **350°F** = 180°C
- **400°F** = 200°C
- **450°F** = 230°C

If your oven only shows one of these units, then understanding how to convert means your baked or roasted foods get to the right temperature.

Length Conversions

Periodically, recipes may state the length or thickness of ingredients, especially doughs or vegetables. Below are useful conversions:

- **1 inch** = 2.54 centimeters (cm)
- **1 centimeter** = 0.39 inches

These conversions are especially useful when you need to slice ingredients to a certain thickness or are working with recipes that provide these details.

Common Ingredient Conversions

Some ingredients have unique densities, which means their weight doesn't always translate evenly. Here's a quick reference for commonly used ingredients:

- **1 cup butter** = 227 grams (g) = 8 ounces (oz)
- **1 cup shredded cheese** = 113 grams (g) = 4 ounces (oz)
- **1 cup rice (uncooked)** = 190 grams (g)

Having specific conversions for items like butter and cheese can be particularly helpful in baking or when working with recipes where texture and consistency matter.

Quick Reference Table

To simplify measurements further, here's a quick reference table of some of the most frequently used conversions:

US Unit Metric Equivalent

1 tsp 5 ml

1 tbsp 15 ml

1 fl oz 30 ml

1 cup 237 ml

1 oz 28 g

1 lb 454 g

Using this table, you can quickly convert your ingredients without needing to rely on detailed calculations.

Tips for Accurate Measuring

When taking measurements for dry foods such as flour, use the scoop and level technique where you dip the measuring cup into the pile of flour and then level the contents with a straight edge rather than slamming the measuring cup into the pile of food. Brown sugar should be hard-packed into the cup. While using spoons, it is advisable to take a small measure of liquids, then use a transparent cup and look at the measurement at eye level.

Why Unit Conversions Matter

Proportions are important in cooking or baking, especially when slight changes in the ratio of the ingredients have a great impact. Using conversions is important in baking because baking involves a measure and balance phenomenon, and halving or doubling a recipe requires accurate measurements. For instance, instead of using cups to measure flour, baked products can be either heavy or dry since using grams is more accurate.

Moreover, if you are baking, converting equals preserving the original flavors and textures from recipes obtained from other countries. This page is a transition between different systems, and you can follow any recipe without much guesswork or alteration.

Organizing a unit conversion page keeps recipes easy and simple to use, making your cooking experience more enjoyable. This page allows for the flexibility to measure each ingredient to the preference of milliliters and grams or ounces and cups. With these conversions, you are allowed to cook freely and precisely, transforming any recipe into a success story.

Conclusion

Ready to Make Weeknight Dinners Effortless and Delicious?

Planning and preparing dinner at home is never easy, especially during a working week, but this book makes weeknight dinners attractive and achievable. Explaining step by step, with useful suggestions and basic recipes, this book will help you realize that cooking healthy meals at home is not only possible but also quite enjoyable. You are now equipped with the recipes and strategies of this book to improve your weeknight experience from boring and unproductive to fun, healthy, and timely. It no longer becomes necessary for one to ORDER a takeaway or purchase processed meals; rather, one should cook delicious homemade meals that are easy to prepare.

All the recipes mentioned here have been designed to provide you with easy and convenient recipes for a working woman. Some can be prepared using a small number of ingredients, and every recipe is simple and can be prepared in a short time. It will also interest you to know that preparing these dishes does not require any sort of special culinary skill set; anyone can prepare these dishes. Educate yourself to seek quality ingredients and learn no-nonsense cooking techniques, and you'll get to prepare tasty meals that your whole family can enjoy.

Setting the Stage for Effortless Weeknight Cooking

First on our list is organization, and this is the reason weeknight dinners should not be a problem. Just having enough stock to keep well, an easy-to-follow meal plan, and the ability to reach for the more commonly used ingredients can dramatically affect the ease with which one prepares the dinner. This book helps you arrange your kitchen in order to make cooking easier and more efficient. Having stocks of basics made available and a straightforward schedule makes dinner time more relaxed and easier.

Using the numerous recipes provided in this book, every recipe comes with a shopping list to enable one to buy all the necessary products at one time. Preparing and listing down everything to be bought lessens going to the grocery store and avoids throwing away unwanted food. Most of the ingredients used can be termed all-purpose since they can be utilized in any other recipe. For instance going for olive oil, garlic, fresh herbs, and spices are flexible seasoners that can be used in a wide range of foods, so you are not stuck with a lot of seasoners.

Embracing Variety with Minimal Effort

People order takeout because they want to have options other than what they cooked at home, and with the recipes here, you won't get bored. Finally, let it be said that this book is packed with meals of various origins around the globe. Whether you are into Italian pasta, Mexican tacos, or Asian stir-fries, there is going to be something for everyone. These seven options are not only both quick and flavorful but also avoid the boredom that can set in when you're cooking at home in the middle of the week but don't want to go out.

It is quite common for the recipes to provide options & swaps to achieve that direction so you can change it according to your ingredients. If you find that a particular vegetable or seasoning is not available, you will be informed of the other that can be used in its place to yield almost the same results. This flexibility leads to the preparation of the recipes being bendable to separate and introduce new tastes to them. For instance, if a recipe suggests that chicken should be used, substitute it with shrimp, and what you have on your hands will be a different meal that does not require a new recipe to be found.

Building Confidence in the Kitchen

Cooking doesn't have to feel like a chore, and this book aims to make it something you genuinely enjoy. With step-by-step instructions and tips for each recipe, you'll build skills along the way that will make cooking feel effortless. The recipes are written to be easy to follow, helping you learn techniques and gain confidence as you go. People order takeout because they want to have options other than what they cooked at home, and with the recipes here, you won't get bored. Finally, let it be said that this book is packed with meals of various origins around the globe. Whether you are into Italian pasta, Mexican tacos, or Asian stir-fries, there is something for everyone. These seven options are not only both quick and flavorful but also avoid the boredom that can set in when you're cooking at home in the middle of the week but don't want to go out.

It is quite common for the recipes to provide options & swaps to achieve that direction so you can change it according to your ingredients. If you find that a particular vegetable or seasoning is not available, you will be informed of the other that can be used in its place to yield almost the same results. This flexibility leads to the preparation of the recipes being bendable to separate and introduce new tastes to them. For instance, if a recipe suggests that chicken should be used, substitute it with shrimp, and what you have on your hands will be a different meal that does not require a new recipe to be found.

Prioritizing Health Without Sacrificing Flavor

Eating well is essential, and these recipes prioritize health without compromising taste. By cooking at home, you have full control over the ingredients that go into your meals, allowing you to make nutritious choices. The recipes are crafted to include fresh vegetables, lean proteins, and wholesome grains, giving you balanced meals that taste fantastic. For those looking to cut back on sugar, salt, or fat, home cooking offers a way to adjust these elements to your liking, ensuring you're nourishing your body with each meal.

With each recipe, nutritional considerations are kept in mind. Many dishes are low in unhealthy fats and sugars, incorporating natural flavors from herbs, spices, and high-quality ingredients instead. This focus on health means you're not just saving time and money but also making choices that benefit your overall well-being. Simple adjustments, like using olive oil instead of butter or opting for whole grains, are suggested throughout the book so you can create meals that align with your health goals without feeling like you're missing out on flavor.

Making Cooking a Stress-Free Part of Your Day

The goal of this book is to make cooking feel less like an obligation and more like a rewarding break in your day. With the right approach, preparing dinner can become a calming, enjoyable experience rather than something to rush through. Following a recipe, focusing on the steps, and putting a meal together can even be a form of relaxation, helping you unwind after a busy day. Knowing that the recipes are simple and reliable means you can focus on the process, trusting that the results will be delicious.

These recipes are meant to fit into real life, understanding that sometimes you need dinner on the table quickly. By keeping preparation times short and steps minimal, the book is designed to accommodate even the busiest schedules. Each recipe is straightforward, allowing you to prepare everything in under 30 minutes so that you can focus on enjoying your meal and the rest of your evening.

Reducing Dependency on Takeout

With the tools and recipes in this book, you're equipped to leave behind the habit of ordering takeout. Homemade meals offer a level of quality and flavor that takeout often lacks, and by cooking at home, you can customize each dish to suit your preferences. Plus, cooking at home is a huge cost-saver; you'll find that the same amount spent on one takeout meal can cover the ingredients for multiple homemade dinners.

Takeout and pre-packaged meals are convenient, but they're often loaded with extra salt, sugar, and preservatives. By cooking at home, you're able to make healthier choices while also exploring a range of flavors that suit your taste. You'll find that the satisfaction of a homemade meal, paired with the health and financial benefits, far outweighs the convenience of takeout.

Enjoying the Process of Cooking and Sharing Meals

Cooking isn't just about making food; it's about creating an experience that brings joy and satisfaction. This book encourages you to enjoy the process, from gathering ingredients to the final plating. Each recipe is a chance to create something special, whether you're cooking for yourself, your family, or your friends. Sharing a meal that you've made yourself is an experience that goes beyond just eating; it's a way to connect, celebrate, and show care.

For families, these recipes provide an opportunity to spend time together, teaching children about cooking or simply gathering around the table for a wholesome, home-cooked meal. Even if you're cooking for one, each dish is crafted to be enjoyable and comforting, bringing a sense of fulfillment and nourishment.

Bringing Pride and Ease to Weeknight Meals

By following this book, you're ready to turn weeknight dinners into an effortless and rewarding part of your life. You'll find that with each recipe, you build a sense of pride and achievement, knowing that you've created something delicious and wholesome. Say goodbye to the hassle of planning last-minute meals or ordering out because now, with these recipes, you're equipped to handle any weeknight dinner with ease.

As you continue to use this book, cooking at home will become second nature, and you'll likely find that it's something you look forward to. With quick, healthy, and flavorful recipes at your fingertips, you're prepared to enjoy the comfort and satisfaction that comes with home-cooked meals. Welcome to a new way of eating and living, where weeknight dinners are effortless, enjoyable, and always delicious.

Made in United States
North Haven, CT
16 January 2025